HEALTH CARE IN TRANSITION

MEDICAID THIRD-PARTY LIABILITY

SAVINGS ISSUES AND EFFORTS

HEALTH CARE IN TRANSITION

Additional books in this series can be found on Nova's website under the Series tab.

Additional e-books in this series can be found on Nova's website under the e-book tab.

HEALTH CARE IN TRANSITION

MEDICAID THIRD-PARTY LIABILITY

SAVINGS ISSUES AND EFFORTS

DONALD MURPHY
EDITOR

nova publishers
New York

NOTICE TO THE READER

Library of Congress Cataloging-in-Publication Data

ISBN: 978-1-63483-049-2

Published by Nova Science Publishers, Inc. † New York

CONTENTS

PREFACE

In fiscal year 2013, Medicaid—jointly financed by states and the federal government—provided health care coverage to over 70 million individuals at a total cost of about $460 billion. Congress generally established Medicaid as the health care payer of last resort, meaning that if enrollees have another source of health care coverage—such as private insurance—that source should pay, to the extent of its liability, before Medicaid does. This is referred to as third-party liability (TPL). There are known challenges to ensuring that Medicaid is the payer of last resort. This book examines the extent to which Medicaid enrollees have private insurance; and state and Centers for Medicare & Medicaid Services (CMS) initiatives to improve TPL efforts. Provided in this book is the Effective Practices Guide. It's intent is to provide state Medicaid agencies with information on practices that could assist states in improving their identification and successful pursuit of legally liable third party resources.

In: Medicaid Third-Party Liability
Editor: Donald Murphy
ISBN: 978-1-63483-049-2

Chapter 1

MEDICAID: ADDITIONAL FEDERAL ACTION NEEDED TO FURTHER IMPROVE THIRD-PARTY LIABILITY EFFORTS*

United States Government Accountability Office

ABBREVIATIONS

ACS	American Community Survey
CHIP	State Children's Health Insurance Program
CMS	Centers for Medicare & Medicaid Services
COB	coordination of benefits
DRA	Deficit Reduction Act of 2005
ERISA	Employee Retirement Income Security Act of 1974
FAQ	Frequently Asked Questions
HHS	Department of Health and Human Services
MHPA	Medicaid Health Plans of America
OIG	Office of Inspector General
PIE	payer initiated eligibility/benefit

* This is an edited, reformatted and augmented version of The United States Government Accountability Office publication, GAO-15-208 , dated January 2015.

PPACA	Patient Protection and Affordable Care Act
PUMS	Public Use Microdata Sample
TAG	technical advisory group
TPL	third-party liability
VA	Department of Veterans Affairs

WHY GAO DID THIS STUDY

In fiscal year 2013, Medicaid—jointly financed by states and the federal government—provided health care coverage to over 70 million individuals at a total cost of about $460 billion. Congress generally established Medicaid as the health care payer of last resort, meaning that if enrollees have another source of health care coverage—such as private insurance—that source should pay, to the extent of its liability, before Medicaid does. This is referred to as third-party liability (TPL). There are known challenges to ensuring that Medicaid is the payer of last resort. GAO was asked to provide information on the prevalence of private insurance among Medicaid enrollees and on state and CMS efforts to ensure that Medicaid is the payer of last resort.

This report examines (1) the extent to which Medicaid enrollees have private insurance, and (2) state and CMS initiatives to improve TPL efforts. GAO analyzed the 2012 ACS; interviewed Medicaid officials from eight states with high program spending or enrollment that used managed care; interviewed CMS officials and stakeholders; and reviewed relevant laws, regulations, and CMS guidance.

WHAT GAO RECOMMENDS

GAO recommends that the Secretary of the Department of Health and Human Services (HHS) direct CMS to

1. routinely monitor and share across all states information regarding key TPL efforts and challenges, and
2. provide guidance on state oversight of TPL efforts conducted by Medicaid managed care plans. HHS concurred with GAO's recommendations and noted plans to address them.

What GAO Found

Based on responses to the 2012 U.S. Census Bureau's American Community Survey (ACS)—the most recent available at the time the work was conducted— GAO estimates that 7.6 million Medicaid enrollees (13.4 percent) had private health insurance in 2012. The estimated prevalence of private health insurance varied among Medicaid eligibility categories, which may differ with respect to Medicaid benefits and costs. The number of Medicaid enrollees with private health insurance is expected to increase with the expansion of Medicaid.

Selected states reported taking various steps to address challenges to ensuring that Medicaid is the payer of last resort and acknowledged recent Centers for Medicare & Medicaid Services (CMS) support, while also suggesting additional federal action. Four of the eight reviewed states reported various initiatives to improve coverage identification, such as arranging to participate in a data registry that allows participants to identify individuals with overlapping coverage. CMS has taken steps to issue TPL guidance and share some information on effective state practices, and such federal efforts should be ongoing to ensure that evolving approaches are captured and shared across states. In addition, officials in five states reported that enrollees with third-party coverage may be eligible to enroll in Medicaid managed care—in which states contract with health plans to provide services to enrollees and may delegate TPL activities such as payment recoveries to these plans. One of the five states had initiated a program to oversee plans' TPL recoveries, while other states did not report similar oversight. The National Association of Medicaid Directors reported that, in the absence of explicit CMS guidance in this area, it can be difficult for states to work with plans to improve TPL oversight and has recommended CMS provide such guidance.

* * *

January 28, 2015

The Honorable Joseph R. Pitts
Chairman
Subcommittee on Health
Committee on Energy and Commerce
House of Representatives

The Honorable Michael C. Burgess, M.D.
House of Representatives

In fiscal year 2013, Medicaid provided health care coverage to over 70 million individuals at a total cost of about $460 billion.[1] Congress generally established Medicaid as the health care payer of last resort, meaning that if Medicaid enrollees have another source of health care coverage, that source should pay, to the extent of its liability, before Medicaid does. Federal regulation refers to this requirement as third-party liability (TPL).[2] In administering their Medicaid programs, states are required to take certain steps to identify sources of third-party coverage that Medicaid enrollees may have, and to ensure that these sources pay to the extent of their liability.[3] When private third parties—such as health insurers—pay for health care services instead of Medicaid, savings accrue not only to states, but also to the federal government, which historically has financed over half of the overall Medicaid program costs.[4] In addition, federal financing of Medicaid is increasing with the implementation of the Patient Protection and Affordable Care Act (PPACA), under which states may expand Medicaid eligibility to certain low-income individuals and which specified that the federal government would pay 100 percent of costs for these individuals from 2014 through 2016, and a minimum of 90 percent of such costs thereafter.[5] Therefore, state efforts to ensure that health insurers pay to the extent of their liability, particularly for Medicaid enrollees who are newly eligible for the program, could lead to increased federal cost savings.

States have substantially improved their TPL identification and recovery efforts (which we refer to hereafter as TPL efforts) in recent years, generating significant savings for the federal government as well as for themselves. A 2013 Department of Health and Human Services (HHS) Office of Inspector General (OIG) report indicated that states identified about $13.6 billion in combined federal-state cost savings from private health insurers in 2011, compared to about $3.7 billion in 2001—with states largely crediting increased cost savings to enhanced use of available technology to identify Medicaid enrollees with other insurance.[6] However, the report also found that states commonly face challenges to their TPL efforts, such as health insurers refusing to provide coverage information to states or denying liability for procedural reasons, that pose potential barriers to realizing cost savings. Furthermore, state Medicaid agencies face administrative capacity constraints that may limit their ability to go beyond basic program requirements to further improve cost savings.[7]

Given the PPACA Medicaid expansion and the importance of ensuring that Medicaid appropriately pays only after other liable third parties have done so, you asked us to examine the prevalence of private sources of health insurance among Medicaid enrollees, and state and Centers for Medicare & Medicaid Services (CMS) efforts to ensure that Medicaid is the payer of last resort. In this report, we examine (1) the extent to which Medicaid enrollees have private health insurance and (2) state and CMS initiatives to improve TPL efforts.

To examine the extent to which Medicaid enrollees have private health insurance, we analyzed 2012 data—the most recent data available at the time we conducted the work—from the American Community Survey (ACS), a nationally representative annual survey conducted by the U.S. Census Bureau. The ACS collects self-reported information, such as each individual's type of health coverage (if any) as of the date of the survey, disability status, age, and state of residence. For the ACS question regarding each individual's type of health coverage, Medicaid is grouped with other types of means-tested public coverage as a single response option.[8] Therefore, for purposes of the report, we refer to these groups collectively as Medicaid enrollees. We further divided Medicaid enrollees into four broad Medicaid eligibility categories—children, adults, disabled, and aged.[9] For all Medicaid enrollees, and for each Medicaid eligibility category, we estimated the number and percentage with private health insurance and other sources of health coverage. We defined individuals as having private health insurance if they reported health insurance provided through an employer or union, or health insurance purchased individually. Unless noted otherwise, estimates presented in this report have a relative standard error of less than 15 percent. To determine the reliability of the ACS data, we reviewed related documentation and compared our results to other published estimates and determined that the ACS data were sufficiently reliable for our purposes. (A more detailed description of our methodology is provided in app. I.)

To examine CMS and state initiatives to improve TPL efforts, we reviewed relevant federal laws, regulations, and related documents, and interviewed officials from CMS and a sample of 8 states. To select the sample of states, we began by identifying states that: (1) were among the top 15 states with respect to either Medicaid enrollment or spending; and (2) used capitated managed care—in which states pay health plans a monthly fee per Medicaid enrollee in exchange for services provided— to deliver services to some or all Medicaid enrollees.[10] We then reviewed challenges states reported in the 2013 HHS OIG report and obtained input from federal officials and stakeholders about related state legislation or practices and selected 8 of these states to include in our review:

Georgia, Massachusetts, Michigan, Minnesota, Missouri, New York, Ohio, and Washington. In several cases, officials in these states asked the contractor responsible for aspects of TPL work in their state to respond to our questions or included contractor representatives in the interviews. To supplement information from the selected states, we also interviewed or reviewed information provided by representatives of HMS—a firm that conducts various TPL services on behalf of over 30 states and about 160 Medicaid managed care plans—national associations representing Medicaid directors and Medicaid managed care plans, and other stakeholders.

We conducted this performance audit from December 2013 through January 2015 in accordance with generally accepted government auditing standards. Those standards require that we plan and perform the audit to obtain sufficient, appropriate evidence to provide a reasonable basis for our findings and conclusions based on our audit objectives. We believe that the evidence obtained provides a reasonable basis for our findings and conclusions based on our audit objectives.

BACKGROUND

Medicaid enrollees across various eligibility categories may have access to private health insurance for a number of reasons. For example, some adults may be covered by employer-sponsored private health insurance even though they also qualify for Medicaid. Children similarly may be eligible for Medicaid while also being covered as a dependent on a parent's private health plan. Individuals age 65 and older may receive private coverage from a former employer or purchase such coverage to supplement their Medicare coverage. Medicaid benefits and costs may vary depending on an enrollee's eligibility category.[11] CMS requires states to provide for the identification of Medicaid enrollees' other sources of health coverage, verification of the extent of the other sources' liability for services, avoidance of payment for services in most circumstances where the state believes a third party is liable, and recovery of reimbursement from liable third parties after Medicaid payment, if the state can reasonably reimbursement.[12] Specifically, states must provide that the following steps are taken:

1. *Coverage identification.* To identify enrollees with third-party health coverage, states are required to request coverage information from potential Medicaid enrollees at the time of any determination or redetermination of eligibility for Medicaid. States are also required to obtain and use information pertaining to third-party liability, for example by conducting data matches with state wage information agencies, Social Security Administration wage and earning files, state motor vehicle accident report files, or state workers compensation files.
2. *Coverage verification.* When other health coverage is identified, states need to verify the information, including the services covered through the other insurance and the dates of eligibility.
3. *Cost avoidance.* Cost avoidance occurs when states do not pay providers for services until any other coverage has paid to the extent of its liability, rather than paying up front and recovering costs later. After a state has verified other coverage, it must generally seek to ensure that health care providers' claims are directed to the responsible party.[13] The cost-avoidance process accounts for the bulk of the cost savings associated with third-party liability.
4. *Payment recovery.* When states have already paid providers for submitted claims for which a third party is liable, they must seek reimbursement from the third party, if it is cost effective to do so.

States have flexibility in determining specific approaches to achieve these ends. For example, states are increasingly contracting with managed care plans to deliver services to Medicaid enrollees (such plans are hereafter referred to as Medicaid managed care plans), and may delegate TPL responsibilities to such plans.[14] Both states and Medicaid managed care plans may obtain the services of a contractor to identify third-party coverage by conducting electronic data matches and to conduct other TPL responsibilities, such as payment recovery.

Ensuring compliance with Medicaid TPL requirements has long been challenging for states. The McCarran-Ferguson Act affirms the authority of states to regulate the business of insurance in the state, without interference from federal regulation, unless federal law specifically provides otherwise.[15] Thus, states generally regulate private health insurers operating in the state. However, states may not have authority over private insurers that are not licensed to do business in the state but still provide coverage to state residents. For example, some individuals work and receive health insurance through employment in one state but live in a neighboring state. In addition, states are preempted by the Employee Retirement Income Security Act of 1974 (ERISA) from regulating employer-sponsored health benefit plans that self-insure coverage rather than purchase coverage from an insurer.[16]

Due to the bifurcated nature of private health insurance regulation, both federal and state legislation has been required to allow states to enforce TPL requirements. For example, the Omnibus Budget Reconciliation Act of 1993 required all states to enact laws prohibiting insurers from taking Medicaid status into account in enrollment or payment for benefits and to enact laws giving the state rights to payments by liable third parties.[17] In addition, the Deficit Reduction Act of 2005 (DRA) contained provisions affecting state authority to verify coverage and recoup payments from liable health insurers. Under the DRA, states must attest that they have laws in place to require health insurers to, among other requirements, provide information necessary to identify Medicaid enrollees with third-party coverage and, within specified time limits, respond to inquiries from the state regarding claims, as well as to agree not to deny claims solely because of the date the claim was submitted, the form that was used, or the failure to properly document coverage at the point of service.[18]

The 2013 HHS OIG report on TPL cost savings and challenges concluded that the DRA provisions likely had a positive effect on states' ability to avoid costs and recover payments from private health insurers, in part through improvements in states' identification of enrollees with insurance. States also credited process improvements, such as online verification of coverage and electronic data matching agreements with private insurers, as well as contractor assistance. However, the study reported that states continue to face key challenges working with private insurers, including the following:

- 96 percent of states reported challenges with insurers denying claims for procedural reasons.
- 90 percent of states reported challenges with insurer willingness to release coverage information to states.
- 86 percent of states reported challenges with insurers providing incomplete or confusing information in response to attempts to verify coverage.
- 84 percent of states reported problems with pharmacy benefit managers—entities which administer pharmacy benefits on behalf of insurers or employers—such as pharmacy benefit managers not

providing coverage information or claiming a lack of authority to pay claims to Medicaid agencies.[19]

AN ESTIMATED 7.6 MILLION MEDICAID ENROLLEES HAD PRIVATE INSURANCE IN 2012 AND THIS NUMBER IS EXPECTED TO INCREASE WITH THE MEDICAID EXPANSION

Based on responses to the U.S. Census Bureau's ACS, we estimate that 7.6 million Medicaid enrollees—13.4 percent—also had a private source of health insurance in 2012.[20] However, the prevalence of private health insurance varied among four Medicaid eligibility categories that we analyzed—children, adults, disabled, and aged. For example, according to our estimates, 34.6 percent of aged Medicaid enrollees also had private health insurance, compared to 12.4 percent of adult Medicaid enrollees and 8.4 percent of children.[21] (See fig. 1 and see app. II, table 1, for more detailed estimates).

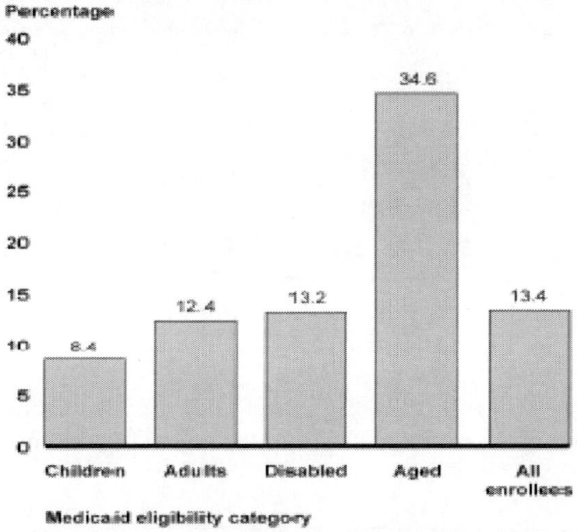

Source: GAO analysis of 2012 U.S. Census Bureau Data. | GAO-15-208.

Notes: Estimates are based on responses to the 2012 American Community Survey (ACS), and have relative standard errors of less than 15 percent. For purposes of this report, the child eligibility category included individuals aged 0 through 18 who did not report a disability; the adult eligibility category included individuals aged 19 through 64 who did not report a disability; the disabled eligibility category included individuals aged 0 through 64 who reported a disability; the aged eligibility category included individuals aged 65 and older

Figure 1. Estimated Prevalence of Private Health Insurance among Medicaid Enrollees by Eligibility Category, 2012.

The number of Medicaid enrollees who also have private health insurance is expected to increase beyond the estimated 7.6 million with the expansion of Medicaid; however, the extent of the increase is uncertain. The Congressional Budget Office projected that approximately 7 million nonelderly individuals would enroll in Medicaid in 2014 as a result of the Medicaid expansion and other PPACA provisions.[22] While some newly Medicaid eligible individuals can be expected to have access to private sources of health insurance, the extent to which they will participate in Medicaid, or maintain private insurance once enrolled in Medicaid, is unknown. If these individuals' rates of private insurance are similar to the 12.4 percent of adult Medicaid enrollees whom we estimated had private insurance in 2012, about 868,000 of the projected 7 million new enrollees in 2014 would be expected to have private insurance.

Selected States Reported Some Success Addressing Challenges to Their TPL Efforts and Additional CMS Action Could Improve Such Efforts Nationwide

States face multiple challenges in ensuring that Medicaid is the payer of last resort for enrollees that have private health insurance. Selected states and CMS have taken various steps to address some of these challenges; however, selected states and stakeholders suggested that further CMS guidance and efforts to facilitate information sharing among states could improve TPL efforts nationwide.

Selected States Have Taken Various Actions to Address Challenges with Coverage Identification, Managed Care Plan TPL Activities, and Coverage Denials

State Actions to Address Challenges with and Improve Coverage Identification

As the identification of Medicaid enrollees with private health insurance is a critical first step for achieving TPL cost savings, many states nationwide conduct electronic data matches of Medicaid enrollment files with insurer files themselves or through a contract with a vendor that conducts matches on the state's behalf. While not required, such state efforts to independently identify enrollees with private insurance can lead to significant cost savings.[23] For example, Minnesota officials reported that by contracting with a vendor for electronic data matching, the state nearly doubled identified cases of TPL in a 5-year period, saving the state an estimated $50 million over this period.[24] Despite such efforts, states we included in our review reported experiencing the following challenges to their coverage identification efforts:

- Challenges obtaining out-of-state coverage data. Medicaid enrollees in one state may have coverage from a health insurer that is licensed in a different state—for example, some enrollees work and participate in employer-sponsored insurance in one state while living and enrolling in Medicaid in a neighboring state. State laws requiring insurers to provide coverage data may not apply if insurers are not licensed in the state, and officials from two of the states we reviewed noted that insurers sometimes refuse to provide coverage data to Medicaid agencies outside the state in which they are licensed. HMS representatives reported that, while HMS advocates that insurers provide coverage data to Medicaid agencies outside the state in which the insurers are licensed, many insurers refuse to do so. According to CMS, there is a significant amount of third-party coverage derived from insurers licensed in a different state from where the Medicaid enrollee resides. [25]
- Challenges with insurers conducting data matches. State and HMS representatives reported that, rather than providing coverage data to the state (or its contractor, as applicable), some insurers request the Medicaid data and perform the data match themselves. HMS representatives reported that, in such cases, states only have access to matches identified by the insurer, which may understate the number of

individuals with overlapping coverage. One state reported estimating that insurers missed the identification of about 7 percent of the individuals with private insurance when insurers conducted the match instead of the state's contractor.

- Challenges with obtaining key data elements. Insurers may not maintain or provide states or their contractors access to key data elements, such as Social Security numbers, and not having access to these data can reduce the efficiency or usefulness of data matches, according to officials in several states we reviewed. For example, officials from two selected states noted that data matches are more difficult and error-prone when Social Security numbers are not available. Similarly, officials from two other states we reviewed reported that their ability to verify identified coverage would be assisted if employer identification numbers were included in insurer coverage data.
- Challenges with timeliness of data matches. Most selected states reported that there is a time lag, typically up to 15 to 30 days, between an individual's enrollment in Medicaid and when the individual is included in a data match with private insurers. As a result, states may not be able to identify other coverage until after enrollees have already begun using services. States would generally then seek reimbursement for paid claims.

States in our review reported taking various steps to address these and other coverage identification challenges. Four of the eight selected states reported initiatives underway or completed to improve data-matching strategies to identify private coverage, some of which focused on nationally coordinated approaches. For example, Minnesota officials reported that Minnesota law allows the state Medicaid agency and Medicaid managed care plans to participate in a national coverage data registry, launched in late 2013 by CAQH, an association of health plans and trade associations.[26] The data registry allows participating insurers and states to submit coverage data files for comparison with files of other participants in order to identify individuals with overlapping coverage. Minnesota officials commented that the registry was at an early stage but expected that participation of private insurers would increase over time because of benefits to private insurers of coordinating with one another. Table 1 describes a variety of initiatives underway or completed to improve coverage data in selected states.

Table 1. Examples of Initiatives in Selected States to Improve Coverage Identification

State	Description of initiative
Massachusetts	The state is in the process of arranging for its vendor to conduct real time data matches—that is, to check for additional insurance at the point that an individual enrolls in Medicaid—which will allow for earlier identification of overlapping coverage. Officials reported aiming for implementation at the end of calendar 2015.
Michigan	The state obtained national coverage data from insurers and developed an in-house, third-party liability (TPL) tracking and billing system, which was implemented in 2006. Officials reported that as a result, cost savings related to TPL had increased exponentially in recent years, and the state was able to reduce its reliance on a vendor to conduct data matches.
Minnesota	The state and Medicaid managed care plans with which it contracts plan to participate in a registry launched by CAQH in late 2013 that allows participating insurers and states to identify individuals with overlapping coverage.Participating insurers submit full national coverage data to be matched against data submitted by all other participants in the registry on a weekly basis. State officials anticipated that the registry could possibly be leveraged to permit identification of TPL at the point of enrollment. State officials anticipated that participation in this registry would begin in early 2015.
Washington	The state implemented a nationally standardized format for receiving coverage data developed by the Centers for Medicare & Medicaid Services (CMS), called the Payer Initiated Eligibility/Benefit (PIE) Transaction. The PIETransaction allows states that elect to adopt it to obtain eligibility information from insurers automatically and allows insurers to set up one standard file to share with any state that had implemented it.

Source: GAO analysis of interviews with selected state officials. | GAO-15-208.

In addition, at least two of the eight states had laws that addressed challenges with obtaining private insurer compliance with TPL requirements, including requirements to provide coverage data. For example, Michigan law authorizes the state to collect coverage data from insurers to determine TPL and to assess penalties on insurers for noncompliance.[27] Michigan officials reported that the state was successful in obtaining national coverage data from insurers. In addition, Minnesota law requires that all insurers that cover state Medicaid enrollees must comply with TPL requirements irrespective of where they are licensed.[28]

State Actions to Support and Oversee Medicaid Managed Care Plan TPL Activities

Selected states have taken various actions that support or increase oversight of Medicaid managed care plan TPL activities, as applicable. For example, in five of the eight states in our review, individuals with third-party coverage may be eligible to enroll in Medicaid managed care plans and certain TPL responsibilities are delegated to these plans.[29] The laws of two selected states—Ohio and Minnesota—specifically authorize Medicaid managed care plans to recover TPL payments on the state's behalf.[30] Ohio officials in particular credited the legislation as effective in improving insurer cooperation with the state's Medicaid managed care plans. While the DRA required states to have laws in effect compelling insurers to provide states with access to data and recognize the states right to recoup payments, it did not provide that those laws specifically require insurers to similarly cooperate with Medicaid managed care plans conducting such work on behalf of states. CMS provided guidance that, when states delegate TPL responsibilities to a Medicaid managed care plan, third-parties should treat the plan as if it were the state.[31] HMS representatives reported that this guidance has been effective in garnering cooperation from insurers that previously refused to provide coverage data or pay claims to Medicaid managed care plans in various states without legislation specifically requiring them to do so. However, a few insurers continue to refuse to cooperate with such plans despite this guidance, according to information provided by representatives of HMS and Medicaid Health Plans of America (MHPA)—an association of Medicaid managed care plans.

In addition, Minnesota sought to improve its oversight of Medicaid managed care TPL activities by initiating a program to allow the state to review Medicaid managed care plan TPL payment recoveries and to arrange for conducting supplemental recoveries when the plans had not recouped payment within a set time.[32] However, according to a representative of the National Association of Medicaid Directors, it can be difficult for states to work with Medicaid managed care plans and insurers as needed to strengthen state oversight. The other states included in our review that delegate TPL work to Medicaid managed care plans did not report conducting this type of oversight, which is consistent with information provided by MHPA in which plans indicated that some states that contract with Medicaid managed care plans to perform TPL activities do not specifically review these activities. We have previously found that some Medicaid managed care plans may have a conflict of interest in conducting payment recoveries. Specifically, Medicaid managed care plans may not have appropriate incentives to identify and recover improper payments—which include payments made for treatments or services that were not covered by program rules, that were not medically necessary, or that were billed for but never provided—because doing so could reduce future capitation rates.[33]

State Actions to Reduce Denials by Insurers for Procedural Reasons

Most selected states reported challenges with denials from private insurers for procedural reasons, such as for not obtaining prior authorization before receiving services or not using in-network providers.[34] HMS representatives estimated that in 2013, insurers had denied about $120 million in claims for failure to obtain prior authorization, and about $30 million for failure to use an in-network provider, for states and for Medicaid managed care plans with which HMS contracted. Selected states reported various methods to reduce such denials:

- Ohio and Missouri laws explicitly prohibit denials due solely to a lack of prior authorization for services.[35]
- Massachusetts, Georgia, and New York officials reported that they contest denials due solely to a lack of prior authorization for services based on general state legislation passed in accordance with the DRA, which requires states to prohibit insurers from denying claims based solely on the date the claim was submitted, the form that was used, or the failure to properly document coverage at the point of service.[36]
- Michigan and Minnesota, through their Medicaid provider manuals, require providers to check for third-party coverage and specify that providers are not to be paid by Medicaid for services provided to enrollees if rules of the third-party coverage were not followed.[37] For example, Michigan's Medicaid provider manual states that Medicaid will not cover charges incurred when enrollees elect to go out of their third-party insurer's preferred provider network. Michigan and Minnesota officials reported that these types of denials were generally not problems for the state.

While CMS Has Taken Action to Support State TPL Efforts, Additional Federal Action Could Benefit TPL Efforts Nationwide

CMS has taken steps, including issuing additional guidance, to address certain challenges that states face in ensuring that Medicaid is the payer of last resort. For example, CMS published a set of frequently asked questions (FAQ) in September 2014 that clarified the parameters under which health insurers are permitted to release coverage information to states in light of Health Insurance Portability and Accountability Act of 1996 privacy restrictions, and emphasized the role of state legislation in specifying the scope of information required to be submitted by health insurers.[38] The guidance also reiterated previously published information, such as clarifying that when states delegate TPL responsibilities to a Medicaid managed care plan, third parties are required to treat the plan as if it were the state.[39] CMS officials also noted that the agency is available to provide technical assistance relating to TPL at the request of states or other entities.

In addition, CMS has also taken steps to foster collaboration among states. For example, CMS solicited effective TPL practices that had been implemented as of 2013 from states and published the responses.[40] On a related note, CMS officials highlighted the role of the Coordination of Benefits (COB)-TPL Technical Advisory Group (TAG) in providing states with opportunities to coordinate and share information on TPL challenges and effective practices.[41] Specifically, CMS officials said that COB-TPL TAG representatives are responsible for canvassing states about problems that may be occurring and reporting these back to CMS. However, officials from one state suggested that COB-TPL TAG representatives need to do more to proactively survey states and share information about problems that states not directly represented on the COB-TPL TAG are experiencing.

While acknowledging CMS's efforts, stakeholders and officials from selected states suggested a need for additional federal action, commenting on how, for example, additional or clarified guidance could facilitate state efforts to conduct certain TPL activities.

- The National Association of Medicaid Directors recommended, given the growth in states' use of managed care, that CMS require states to share available insurance coverage information with Medicaid managed care plans and provide an approved approach for conducting oversight of such plans' TPL activities. According to a representative of this association, several states indicated that explicit CMS guidance in this area would provide states leverage to strengthen their Medicaid managed care plan contracts and oversight related to TPL.

- HMS representatives recommended that CMS strengthen its statements encouraging insurers to share coverage information with out-of-state Medicaid agencies, and further clarify through regulations existing CMS guidance regarding insurer cooperation with Medicaid managed care plans that conduct TPL activities on behalf of states.
- State officials suggested that CMS could provide information to ensure all states are aware of promising available data-matching strategies.

CMS, however, may have incomplete information to inform such guidance as, according to CMS, the agency does not actively track all states' coverage-identification strategies on an ongoing basis, and in some cases, may not be aware of promising state initiatives. While the effective state practices CMS solicited and shared with states included information on initiatives implemented as of 2013, other state initiatives underway were not included. For example, Minnesota officials said they had submitted information about the CAQH data registry; however, the state's submission did not meet the criteria for inclusion in the effective practices document because the state had not yet implemented the registry. In addition, while CMS suggests that states should oversee Medicaid managed care plan TPL activities, as applicable, the agency does not track which states delegate TPL responsibilities to Medicaid managed care plans, nor the problems with or oversight of related Medicaid managed care plan TPL activities in states that do.

Officials from selected states also emphasized efficiencies and other benefits that could be gained from state collaboration and information sharing, which CMS could support. For example, Michigan officials noted that the state wanted to explore sharing the national coverage data it obtained from insurers, as well as the TPL tracking and billing system it developed, with other states, noting the cost-effectiveness of states using its system and data rather than each developing their own. In addition, officials in multiple states noted the value of CMS-facilitated national TPL conferences that provide states with opportunities to discuss emerging problems and share expertise regarding solutions.[42] CMS officials indicated that the last conference occurred when there were significant changes under the DRA and that CMS has no specific plans to facilitate future TPL conferences, but officials noted that discussions were underway regarding additional conferences or other training opportunities.

CONCLUSION

National survey data suggest that a substantial number of Medicaid enrollees—7.6 million—had private health insurance in 2012 and that many of these enrollees were in eligibility groups that incur, traditionally, higher medical costs. Furthermore, this number is expected to increase because of the Medicaid expansion. States have front-line responsibility for ensuring that Medicaid is the payer of last resort and are required to take steps to identify individuals with other health insurance and ensure that other insurance pays to the extent of its liability. Substantial increases in TPL cost savings in recent years highlight that improvements to TPL efforts, such as heightened attention to coverage identification, can substantially improve TPL cost avoidance and recoveries. The scale of the cost savings to Medicaid at both federal and state levels through the identification of coverage through, and payment of services by, private health insurance—reportedly nearly $14 billion in 2011—underscores the potentially significant return on investment that may be gained from continued TPL improvement efforts and attention to resolving remaining gaps in state access to available coverage data.

Selected states have taken a variety of steps to further improve TPL efforts, and other states may also be implementing initiatives to address persistent challenges states report in ensuring Medicaid pays after other liable third parties. The various initiatives that selected states have undertaken—such as initiatives to improve identification of enrollees with private health insurance through data matches or to ensure that TPL efforts are maintained in an increasingly managed care environment— highlight options that other states could consider to improve their respective TPL savings. Other states may also have initiatives that could be adopted more broadly. CMS has taken steps to support states and publicize effective state practices. However, as new strategies emerge over time, a robust ongoing effort to collect and share information about state initiatives would ensure that states—particularly any states that may not conduct data matches with private insurers— are aware of available data matching strategies and solutions to challenges states or Medicaid managed care plans may face in conducting TPL activities. Given the significant federal Medicaid outlays, which are increasing as Medicaid expands under PPACA, the federal government has a vested financial interest in further increasing states' TPL cost savings, and CMS should play a more active leadership role in monitoring, understanding, supporting and promoting state TPL efforts.

RECOMMENDATIONS

In light of the federal interest in ensuring that Medicaid should pay only after other liable third parties; state initiatives to improve TPL efforts, such as coverage identification strategies; and states' increasing use of managed care, we recommend that the Secretary of Health and Human Services direct CMS to take the following two additional actions to oversee and support state TPL efforts:

- Routinely monitor and share across all states information regarding key TPL efforts and challenges.
- Provide guidance to states on their oversight of TPL efforts conducted by Medicaid managed care plans.

AGENCY COMMENTS

We provided a draft of this report to HHS for comment. In its written comments HHS concurred with our recommendations. HHS stated that it will continue to look at ways to provide guidance to states to allow for sharing of effective practices and to increase awareness of initiatives under development in states. HHS also stated that it will explore the need for additional guidance regarding state oversight of TPL efforts conducted by Medicaid managed care plans.

Katherine M. Iritani, Director, Health Care

APPENDIX I: SCOPE AND METHODOLOGY OF THE AMERICAN COMMUNITY SURVEY (ACS) ANALYSIS

To assess the extent to which Medicaid enrollees have private health insurance, we utilized the ACS, an annual survey conducted by the U.S.

Census Bureau. The ACS includes representative samples of households from each state and also includes individuals residing in institutions such as nursing homes. The ACS collects self-reported information, such as the type of health insurance coverage as of the date of the survey (if any), disability status, age, and state of residence. We analyzed data from the most recent ACS Public Use Microdata Sample (PUMS) that was available at the time we conducted our work, which covered calendar year 2012.[1]

Our analysis of ACS PUMS data is subject to limitations. The analysis uses 2012 data and therefore does not include individuals who were newly eligible for Medicaid in 2014 as a result of the optional program expansion under the Patient Protection and Affordable Care Act. In addition, our estimates are based on responses from the ACS PUMS sample and may differ from actual figures that would be obtained if the full population had been surveyed using the same methods. Similarly, as the ACS collects self-reported information, errors may exist due to factors such as differing interpretations of survey questions, the inability or unwillingness of survey participants to provide correct information, or data processing errors. The Census Bureau reported that quality control and edit procedures were used to reduce such errors. For example, an eligibility edit was applied to assign Medicaid, Medicare, and TRICARE coverage to individuals based on program eligibility rules.[2] To determine the reliability of the ACS PUMS data, we reviewed related documentation and compared the results to estimates based on data from another Census Bureau survey, the Current Population Survey. We determined that the ACS PUMS data were sufficiently reliable for the purposes of our engagement.

KEY ANALYSIS VARIABLES

From the available ACS PUMS data, we constructed the following variables for our analysis:

- *Medicaid coverage and eligibility category*. We defined individuals as having Medicaid if they reported health coverage through Medicaid, medical assistance, or any kind of government assistance plan for individuals with low incomes or a disability. These sources of coverage are combined in one question in the ACS PUMS.[3] For purposes of the report, we refer to these individuals collectively as Medicaid enrollees.

We further categorized Medicaid enrollees into four broad Medicaid eligibility categories—children, adults, disabled, and aged:

- We defined the child eligibility category as individuals aged 0 through 18 who did not report a disability.
- We defined adult eligibility category as individuals aged 19 through 64 who did not report a disability.
- We defined the disabled eligibility category as individuals aged 0 through 64 who reported one or more of the 6 disability indicators included in the ACS data.[4]
- We defined the aged eligibility category as individuals aged 65 and older.
- Third-party private and public health coverage. We defined individuals as having private insurance coverage if they reported having health insurance through a current or former employer or union, insurance purchased directly from an insurance company, or both. We defined individuals as having public coverage other than Medicaid if they reported coverage through Medicare or TRICARE, or having ever used or enrolled in health care provided through the Department of Veterans Affairs (VA).[5]

METHODOLOGY

Based on the variables defined above, we used calendar year 2012 ACS PUMS data to estimate the number and percentage of Medicaid enrollees with private and other sources of health coverage. We produced separate estimates by Medicaid eligibility group and state of residence. To generate our estimates, we applied the appropriate weights contained in the ACS PUMS data files in order to expand the sample to represent the total population and to account for the complex sample design. Specifically, we used the person weights to generate estimated numbers and percentages.[6] We used the person replicate weights to generate standard errors.

To assess the precision of our estimates, we calculated a relative standard error for each estimate. A relative standard error is calculated by dividing the standard error of the estimate by the estimate itself. For example, if an estimate has a mean of 100 and a standard error of 20, the relative standard error would be 20/100, which would be 20 percent. Estimates with small relative standard errors are considered more reliable than estimates with large relative standard errors. A small relative standard error is a more precise measurement since there is less variance around the mean. Unless otherwise noted, estimates included in this report have relative standard errors of less than 15 percent.

APPENDIX II: DETAILED ESTIMATES OF MEDICAID ENROLLEES WITH OTHER SOURCES OF HEALTH COVERAGE

The following tables provide more detailed information about the estimates derived from of our analysis of the 2012 American Community Survey (ACS) Public Use Microdata Sample (PUMS). Specifically, tables 1 and 2 provide estimates of the number and percentage of Medicaid enrollees with other sources of health coverage by Medicaid eligibility category and by state.

Table 2. Estimated Number and Percentage of Medicaid Enrollees with Other Private or Public Sources of Health Coverage in 2012, by Eligibility Category

			Medicaid eligibility category[a]		
Source of coverage	Children	Adults	Disabled	Aged	All categories
Private[b]	2,254,373 (8.44%)	1,664,062 (12.39%)	1,276,605 (13.23%)	2,363,891 (34.60%)	7,558,931(13.35%)
Medicare[c]	178,071 (0.67%)	855,302 (6.37%)	2,646,272 (27.42%)	6,831,506 (100%)	10,511,151(18.56%)
TRICARE[d]	156,862 (0.59%)	135,644 (1.01%)	123,540 (1.28%)	319,184 (4.67%)	735,230(1.30%)
Department of Veterans Affairs (VA)[e]	23,948 (0.09%)	155,347 (1.16%)	190,109 (1.97%)	471,094 (6.90%)	840,498(1.48%)
No other coverage	24,203,047 (90.58%)	10,952,795 (81.56%)	6,040,083 (62.59%)	0 (0.00%)	41,195,925(72.75%)

Source: GAO analysis of 2012 U.S. Census Bureau data. | GAO-15-208

Notes: Estimates are based on self-reported information from the American Community Survey (ACS) Public Use Microdata Sample (PUMS) dataset. Individuals may report multiple sources of health coverage. For example, an enrollee may report Medicaid, Medicare, and private coverage. Therefore, estimated numbers for each eligibility category may sum to greater than the total number of enrollees, and estimated percentages may sum to greater than 100 percent. All estimates shown have relative standard errors of less than 15 percent.

[a] We categorized Medicaid enrollees into four broad Medicaid eligibility categories—children (individuals aged 0 through 18 who did not report a disability), adults (individuals aged 19 through 64 who did not report a disability), disabled (individuals aged 0 through 64 who reported a disability), and aged (individuals aged 65 and older).

[b] We defined private sources of health insurance to include employer- or union-sponsored and individually purchased health insurance.

[c] Medicare is a federal health insurance program for individuals aged 65 and older or with certain disabilities and individuals with end-stage renal disease.

[d] TRICARE is a health program operated by the Department of Defense generally for active duty personnel and their dependents, and retirees and their dependents and survivors.

[e] VA provides health care generally for persons who served in active military duty and who were discharged or released under conditions other than dishonorable. In the ACS PUMS, individuals who have ever used or enrolled in VA health care are included in this category.

Table 3. Estimated Number and Percentage of Medicaid Enrollees with Other Private or Public Health Coverage in 2012, by State

	Type of additional coverage			
State	*Private*[a]		*Public*[b]	
Alabama	148,707	15.93 %	221,293	23.71 %
Alaska	15,418 [c]	13.87	21,307	19.17
Arizona	145,995	11.37	196,618	15.31
Arkansas	73,411	11.69	138,000	21.97
California	808,909	10.56	1,384,444	18.07
Colorado	101,233	12.93	138,385	17.68
Connecticut	91,340	14.30	127,763	20.00
Delaware	34,832	18.36	33,802	17.81
District of Columbia	26,258	15.62	29,433	17.50
Florida	381,354	11.23	801,696	23.60
Georgia	214,039	12.52	339,391	19.85
Hawaii	33,903	14.30	43,251	18.25
Idaho	43,127	17.11	46,407	18.41
Illinois	275,647	11.87	357,409	15.39
Indiana	154,077	14.98	191,184	18.59
Iowa	116,280	22.54	121,483	23.55
Kansas	68,438	17.41	82,946	21.10

Table 3. (Continued)

	Type of additional coverage			
State	*Private*[a]		*Public*[b]	
Kentucky	111,051	13.51	188,333	22.91
Louisiana	120,964	11.70	197,423	19.10
Maine	48,732	15.53	77,923	24.83
Maryland	133,520	14.81	162,353	18.01
Massachusetts	241,265	16.38	298,749	20.29
Michigan	332,911	17.11	368,583	18.95
Minnesota	118,720	15.05	141,811	17.98
Mississippi	76,244	10.47	157,527	21.63
Missouri	115,410	12.17	196,883	20.76
Montana	23,543	15.24	33,277	21.55
Nebraska	38,139	15.86	55,229	22.97
Nevada	54,776	16.31	68,847	20.50
New Hampshire	28,746	17.85	38,175	23.71
New Jersey	184,708	14.48	282,584	22.16
New Mexico	52,755	11.11	79,717	16.79
New York	599,711	13.46	817,949	18.36
North Carolina	211,977	12.13	357,624	20.47
North Dakota	13,232	20.59	20,226	31.47
Ohio	298,374	14.76	371,395	18.37
Oklahoma	84,954	12.78	118,692	17.86
Oregon	115,430	16.84	128,846	18.79
Pennsylvania	390,012	17.83	461,480	21.09
Rhode Island	33,356	17.78	50,650	27.01
South Carolina	112,300	12.85	184,120	21.08
South Dakota	20,869	16.80	29,197	23.51
Tennessee	164,825	13.46	251,776	20.55
Texas	466,512	9.99	779,806	16.69
Utah	64,392	19.55	55,008	16.70
Vermont	24,169	15.88	31,576	20.74
Virginia	130,910	14.38	200,777	22.06
Washington	174,679	16.09	217,385	20.03
West Virginia	46,548	13.94	79,360	23.77
Wisconsin	176,384	17.99	195,305	19.92
Wyoming	15,845	20.60	20,019	26.02

Source: GAO analysis of 2012 U.S. Census Bureau data. | GAO-15-208

Notes: Estimates are based on self-reported information from the American Community Survey (ACS) Public Use Microdata Sample (PUMS) dataset. Individuals may report multiple sources of health coverage. For example, an enrollee may report Medicaid, Medicare, and private coverage. Therefore, estimated numbers for each state may sum to greater than the total number of enrollees in the state, and estimated percentages may sum to greater than 100 percent. Estimates shown have relative standard errors of less than 15 percent unless otherwise noted.

[a] We defined private sources of health insurance to include employer- or union-sponsored and individually purchased health insurance.

[b] We defined public sources of coverage to include coverage through Medicare, TRICARE, or the Department of Veterans Affairs (VA). Medicare is a federal health insurance program for individuals aged 65 and older or with certain disabilities and individuals with end-stage renal disease. TRICARE is a health program operated by the Department of Defense generally for active duty military personnel and their dependents and retirees and their dependents and survivors. VA provides health care generally for persons who served in active military duty and who were discharged or released under conditions other than dishonorable. In the ACS PUMS, individuals who have ever used or enrolled in VA health care are included in this category.

[c] The relative standard error of the estimate is 15.6 percent.

End Notes

[1] See Medicaid and State Children's Health Insurance Program (CHIP) Payment and Access Commission, Report to the Congress on Medicaid and CHIP, March 2014 (Washington, D.C.: March 14, 2014). Medicaid is jointly financed by the federal government and states.

[2] See 42 C.F.R. §§ 433.135 et seq. (2013).

[3] States administer their individual Medicaid programs subject to approval and oversight by the Centers for Medicare & Medicaid Services (CMS), a federal agency within the Department of Health and Human Services (HHS).

[4] This report focuses on private health insurance. Under federal regulations, private insurance includes commercial insurance companies offering insurance to individuals or groups, prepaid plans offering medical services or payment for services covered by Medicaid, and organizations administering insurance plans for professional organizations, unions, fraternal groups, employer-employee benefit plans, and other similar organizations, including self-insured and self-funded plans. See 42 C.F.R. § 433.136 (2013). Besides private health insurance, other sources of third-party payment include Medicare, which provides health coverage for individuals aged 65 and over or with certain disabilities and individuals with end-stage renal disease; TRICARE, the health care program generally for active duty military personnel and their dependents, and retirees and their dependents and survivors; and the Department of Veterans Affairs (VA), which provides health care generally for qualifying veterans.

[5] Pub. L. No. 111- 148, §§ 2001 and 10201(c), 124 Stat. 119, 271, 918 (2010), as amended by the Health Care and Education Reconciliation Act, Pub. L. No. 111-152, § 1201, 124 Stat. 1029, 1051 (2010). Under PPACA, states may expand Medicaid eligibility under their state plans to nonpregnant, nonelderly adults who are not eligible for Medicare and whose income does not exceed 133 percent of the federal poverty level. PPACA also imposes a 5

percent income disregard when calculating modified adjusted gross income, which in effect, raises this income limit to 138 percent of the federal poverty level. We refer to state expansion under this authority as the Medicaid expansion. As of July 2014, 26 states and the District of Columbia had opted to expand their Medicaid programs.

[6] HHS Office of Inspector General, Medicaid Third-Party Liability Savings Increased, but Challenges Remain, OEI-05-11-00130 (January 2013). State-reported, inflation-adjusted cost savings increased from about $34 billion in 2001 to about $72 billion in 2011, with the majority of the overall cost savings attributable to cost avoidance and payment recoveries from Medicare. However, there are methodological limitations of the cost savings figures reported by states. For example, states may use various methods to calculate cost savings, and some forms of cost avoidance, such as when a provider directly bills a third party rather than Medicaid, are not possible for states to capture or report.

[7] Limitations in states' administrative capacities are discussed in more detail in a recent Medicaid and CHIP Payment and Access Commission report. For example, see Medicaid and CHIP Payment and Access Commission, Report to the Congress on Medicaid and CHIP, June 2014 (Washington, D.C.: June 13, 2014).

[8] The ACS question combines Medicaid coverage with other types of means-tested public coverage, such as health coverage through any kind of government assistance plan for individuals with low incomes or a disability. Therefore, some individuals we identified as Medicaid enrollees may have other types of means-tested coverage, such as CHIP coverage. While it is not possible to differentiate these groups in ACS data, Medicaid is the largest means-tested program, with over 70 million individuals enrolled during fiscal year 2012.

[9] We defined the child eligibility category as individuals aged 0 through 18 who did not report a disability, we defined the adult eligibility category as individuals aged 19 through 64 who did not report a disability, we defined the disabled eligibility category as individuals aged 0 through 64 who reported a disability, and we defined the aged eligibility category as individuals aged 65 and older.

[10] We included state use of managed care as part of our selection criteria to ensure our review included specific considerations related to conducting TPL efforts in a managed care environment.

[11] For example, we previously estimated that, in 2008, average state per enrollee Medicaid spending varied across eligibility categories, ranging from $2,973 for the child category to $17,609 for the aged category and $19,135 for the disabled category. See GAO, Medicaid: Assessment of Variation among States in Per-Enrollee Spending, GAO-14-456 (Washington, D.C.: June 16, 2014).

[12] See 42 C.F.R. §§ 433.137—433.139 (2013).

[13] Exceptions include claims for prenatal or pediatric services or when coverage is through a parent whose obligation to pay for medical support is enforced by the state's child enforcement agency. See 42 C.F.R. § 433.139(b)(2),(3) (2013).

[14] Alternatively, states may retain TPL responsibilities for individuals in managed care, or they may elect not to enroll individuals with identified TPL in managed care, among other options.

[15] Pub. L. No. 79-15, ch. 20, § 2, 59 Stat. 33, 34 (1945) (codified as amended at 15 U.S.C. § 1012).

[16] 29 U.S.C. § 1144(a). This ERISA preemption therefore results in a different regulatory framework depending on whether the employer purchases its health care coverage from an insurer, which the state regulates, or self-funds its health plan, avoiding many state regulations.

[17] Pub. L. No. 103-66, § 13622, 107 Stat. 312, 632.

[18] Pub. L. No. 109-171, § 6035, 120 Stat. 4, 78 (2006).

[19] See OEI-05-11-00130. Prior GAO and HHS-OIG reports also identified similar challenges. See GAO, Medicaid Third-Party Liability: Federal Guidance Needed to Help States Address Continuing Problems. GAO-06-862 (Washington, D.C.: Sept. 15, 2006) and HHS OIG, Medicaid Recovery of Pharmacy Payments From Liable Third Parties, OEI03-00-00030 (August 2001).

[20] Our estimates of the extent to which individuals with Medicaid have private insurance are relatively consistent with older available estimates. For example, we estimated, based on responses to the 2010 ACS, that about 14 percent of individuals with Medicaid had private insurance in 2010. Similarly, we reported in 2006 that 13 percent of individuals enrolled in Medicaid for an entire year had private insurance at some point during the year, based on an analysis of a separate data source that covered 2002 to 2004. See GAO-06-862.

[21] In addition to private insurance, Medicaid enrollees may also have public health coverage through federal programs such as Medicare or veterans health programs. For example, we estimate that about 18.6 percent of Medicaid enrollees in 2012 also had coverage through Medicare. This report focuses on private sources of third-party coverage, but we provide more detailed estimates of various additional sources of coverage in appendix II.

[22] See Congressional Budget Office, Updated Estimates of the Effects of the Insurance Coverage Provisions of the Affordable Care Act, April 2014. This number includes CHIP enrollees, and was projected to increase to approximately 13 million by 2018. These estimates reflect that states are permitted but not required to expand Medicaid.

[23] Such efforts can be important because Medicaid applicants may not be aware of or report other insurance. Additionally, Medicaid enrollees who do not have other insurance when they first enroll may obtain it later. Some state officials also noted potential concerns about the completeness of self-reported insurance information obtained during new online application procedures—underscoring that the importance of independently obtaining coverage information may be increasing.

[24] While contracting with a vendor to conduct data matches can be beneficial, some states noted limitations with this approach. For example, Minnesota officials noted that the national coverage database maintained by its vendor does not necessarily contain information on all insurers in the state.

[25] CMS guidance highlights the need for states to request that insurers provide coverage data on individuals covered in other states. See CMS, Medicaid and CHIP FAQs: Identification of Medicaid Beneficiaries' Third-Party Resources and Coordination of Benefits with Medicaid (Baltimore, Md.: Sept. 11, 2014). HMS representatives reported that when insurers do not share this data with out-of-state Medicaid agencies or Medicaid managed care plans, it is difficult for HMS to reliably identify or bill for otherwise recoverable out-of-state TPL recoveries on behalf of those state Medicaid agencies or plans.

[26] See Minn. Stat. § 256.01, subdivision 18a (2014).

[27] Mich. Comp. Laws §§ 550.283, 550.287 (2014).

[28] Specifically, the statute imposes these requirements "as a condition of doing business in Minnesota or providing coverage to residents of Minnesota" who are enrollees in state medical programs. See Minn. Stat. § 62A.045 (2014). Although Minnesota officials were not aware of their contractor experiencing significant problems accessing coverage data from insurers licensed in other states, they reported difficulty in collecting payments from a large out-of-state insurer under this statute. Officials said they had asked their contractor to

begin providing reports of insurers that refuse to cooperate with either providing data or paying claims.

[29] Officials in the other three selected states said that the state generally does not enroll Medicaid enrollees with known private insurance in Medicaid managed care plans.

[30] See Ohio Rev. Code § 5160.40(B) (2014) and Minn. Stat. § 62A.045(c) (2014).

[31] CMS had provided this clarification on its website and also included the information in a set of frequently asked questions (FAQ) published in September 2014. See CMS, Medicaid and CHIP FAQs: Identification of Medicaid Beneficiaries' Third-Party Resources.

[32] Minn. Stat. § 256B.69, subdivision 34 (2014).

[33] We recommended that CMS increase its oversight of program integrity efforts, in part through updating its guidance on Medicaid managed care plan program integrity. See GAO, Medicaid Program Integrity: Increased Oversight Needed to Ensure Integrity of Growing Managed Care Expenditures, GAO-14-341. (Washington, D.C.: May 19, 2014). These concerns about incentives could similarly apply to identifying and recovering payments for services from liable third-parties.

[34] Private health plans may place certain conditions on their coverage of services. For example, an insurer may require enrollees to obtain services from providers that are within its provider network, and it may require enrollees to obtain prior authorization before obtaining covered services. When enrollees do not follow these procedures, insurers may deny payment for services that would have been covered had the conditions been met.

[35] See Ohio Rev. Code § 5160.40(A) (2014) and Mo. Rev. Stat. § 208.215.1(1) (2013).

[36] We did not independently assess whether denials due to lack of prior authorization for services are prohibited under the DRA. HMS representatives, however, commented that it is difficult and inefficient to address such denials in states without more specific statutory prohibitions against them.

[37] See Michigan Medicaid Provider Manual, Coordination of Benefits, §§ 1.3, 2.1 (October 2014) and Minnesota Medicaid Provider Manual, Billing Policy (Overview), Section on Coordination of Services (September 2014) and Medicare and Other Insurance, Section on Third-Party Liability (TPL) (December 2013).

[38] See CMS, Medicaid and CHIP FAQs: Identification of Medicaid Beneficiaries' Third-Party Resources.

[39] These CMS FAQs also provided guidance on additional issues noted in the 2013 HHS OIG report on TPL. For example, CMS clarified that states must require insurers to either authorize pharmacy benefit managers or other entities with which they contract to provide coverage information to states, or to provide coverage information directly to states without such entities' assistance.

[40] See CMS, Coordination of Benefits and Third-Party Liability (COB/TPL) in the Medicaid Program: A Guide to Effective State Agency Practices, (Baltimore, Md.: July 2014). Ten states submitted responses, including some of our selected states. For example, Washington officials submitted information about implementation of the PIE Transaction, and Ohio officials submitted information about a state law prohibiting denials based on lack of prior authorization for services.

[41] The COB-TPL TAG includes CMS officials, a state chair, and 10 state representatives, which represent the other states in their respective CMS regions (CMS divides the United States into 10 geographic regions). CMS and state officials also reported that a listserv run by states without CMS involvement is a channel for state communication and collaboration.

[42] States may share TPL information though other avenues that are not necessarily specifically focused on TPL. For example, New York officials reported sharing TPL-related information

with other states at a Medicaid program integrity conference, and at the Medicaid Integrity Institute—a national Medicaid program integrity training program. While federal program integrity efforts center on combating provider fraud, waste, and abuse, some states include TPL under the umbrella of program integrity activities.

End Notes for Appendix I

[1] The ACS PUMS dataset contains a sample of actual responses to the ACS, as well as variables that were constructed based on responses. The ACS PUMS file for 2012 contains data on approximately one percent of the U.S. population.

[2] Medicare is a federal health insurance program for individuals aged 65 and older or with certain disabilities and individuals with end-stage renal disease. TRICARE is a federal health program generally for active-duty military personnel and their dependents, and retirees and their dependents and survivors. Medicaid coverage was assigned to foster children, certain individuals receiving Supplementary Security Income or Public Assistance, and the spouses and children of certain Medicaid beneficiaries. Medicare coverage was assigned to individuals aged 65 and older who received Social Security or Medicaid benefits. TRICARE was assigned to active-duty military personnel and their spouses and children.

[3] Because the ACS PUMS variable combines Medicaid coverage with other types of public coverage, some individuals we identified as Medicaid enrollees may have other types of means-tested coverage, such as Children's Health Insurance Program coverage.

[4] These indicators were (1) self-care difficulty, (2) hearing difficulty, (3) vision difficulty, (4) independent living difficulty, (5) ambulatory difficulty, and (6) cognitive difficulty.

[5] VA provides health care generally for veterans who served in active military duty and who were discharged or released under conditions other than dishonorable. We did not include Indian Health Service coverage as a third-party source of coverage because when individuals have both Medicaid and Indian Health Service coverage, Indian Health Service is the payer of last resort. See 42 C.F.R. § 136.61.

[6] The ACS PUMS data includes survey weights in order to allow users to generate accurate estimates and standard errors from the sample data. The ACS PUMS contains person weights and household weights; person weights are used to generate estimates that pertain to individuals, and household weights are used to generate estimates pertaining to housing units and households. Person and household replicate weights are used to generate accurate standard errors for estimates pertaining to individuals or households respectively.

In: Medicaid Third-Party Liability
Editor: Donald Murphy

ISBN: 978-1-63483-049-2

Chapter 2

MEDICAID THIRD-PARTY LIABILITY SAVINGS INCREASED, BUT CHALLENGES REMAIN*

Office of Inspector General

EXECUTIVE SUMMARY: MEDICAID THIRD-PARTY LIABILITY SAVINGS INCREASED, BUT CHALLENGES REMAIN OEI-05-11-00130

Why We Did This Study

Millions of Medicaid beneficiaries have additional health insurance through third-party sources. If beneficiaries have another source of payment, that source should pay before Medicaid does, up to the extent of its liability. Prior studies from the Office of Inspector General and the Government Accountability Office reported that State Medicaid agencies (States) encountered challenges getting third parties to pay when they are responsible, leading to hundreds of millions of dollars in potential losses each year. To address these challenges, the Deficit Reduction Act of 2005 contained

* This is an edited, reformatted and augmented version of report, OEI-05-11-00130, issued by the Department of Health and Human Services, January 2013.

provisions designed to enhance States' ability to identify and recover payments from liable third parties.

How We Did This Study

We determined trends in Medicaid third-party liability (TPL) savings from 2001 to 2011 by analyzing data that States reported to the Centers for Medicare & Medicaid Services (CMS). We also collected data from States on the amount of money at risk of not being recovered. Finally, we surveyed States regarding factors that (1) helped them save money that third parties should pay and (2) made saving money challenging.

What We Found

Medicaid TPL savings increased; however, $4 billion remains at risk of not being recovered. States' reported savings from cost avoidance drove the growth in TPL savings, although savings from recoveries also contributed. States reported that improvements to their processes facilitated savings. Despite these improvements, States reported longstanding challenges with third parties when trying to identify insurance coverage and recover payments. In addition, States reported challenges—caused, they say, by laws and regulations—that hinder the recovery of payments.

What We Recommend

Since 2001, States have made sizable gains in TPL savings. Improved State processes and congressional action seem to have had some effect. However, a significant amount of money remains at risk of not being recovered. On the basis of the amount of money that is at risk and the longstanding challenges that States continue to face, we recommend that CMS: (1) work with States to address longstanding challenges related to identification of insurance coverage and recovery of payments, (2) address States' challenges with 1-year timely filing limits for Medicare and TRICARE, and (3) work to strengthen enforcement mechanisms designed to deal with uncooperative third parties. CMS concurred with our recommendations.

OBJECTIVES

1. To determine trends in State Medicaid agencies' cost-avoided amounts and amounts recovered through pay and chase from 2001 to 2011.
2. To describe factors that influenced State Medicaid agencies' ability to maximize cost avoidance.
3. To describe factors that influenced State Medicaid agencies' ability to maximize payments recovered through pay and chase and to estimate the amount of money that remains at risk of not being recovered.

BACKGROUND

Millions of Medicaid beneficiaries have additional health insurance through third-party sources. For example, from 2008 to 2010, an estimated 15 percent (approximately 6.8 million) of Medicaid beneficiaries had employer-sponsored health insurance annually.[1] During this same period, an estimated 14 percent (approximately 6.3 million) of beneficiaries had Medicare.[2] Prior studies by OIG and the Government Accountability Office (GAO) reported that States encountered challenges to identifying and recovering payments from third parties, leading to hundreds of millions of dollars in potential losses each year.[3, 4] To address these challenges, the Deficit Reduction Act of 2005 (DRA) contained provisions designed to enhance State Medicaid agencies' (States) ability to identify and obtain payments from liable third parties.

Medicaid Third-Party Liability

Medicaid is intended to be the payer of last resort.[5, 6] If Medicaid beneficiaries have another source of payment for health services or items covered by Medicaid, that source should pay before Medicaid does, up to the extent of its liability. These other sources of payment are referred to as third parties.

Third parties include health insurers; self-insured plans; group health plans; Government-sponsored health insurance, such as Medicare and TRICARE; service benefit plans; managed care organizations; pharmacy benefit managers; and other parties that are, by statute, contract, or agreement, legally responsible for payment of a claim for a health care item or service.[7] CMS interprets other parties to include third-party administrators, fiscal intermediaries, and managed care contractors that administer benefits on behalf of the risk-bearing plan sponsor.[8] Further, CMS includes medical support from absent parents, automobile insurance, workers' compensation, and probate-estate recoveries as third parties.[9]

To ensure that Medicaid does not pay for services for which third parties are liable, States conduct a number of coordination of benefits activities. They include identifying liable third parties, preventing payment on claims for which third parties are liable, and recovering reimbursements from liable third parties.

Identifying Third Parties

Identifying third parties is the first step to ensuring that they pay claims for which they are liable. Federal law requires States to take reasonable measures to identify liable third parties that are responsible for payment of claims for health care items or services.[10] Part of identifying potentially liable third parties is verifying coverage. States must ask beneficiaries at the time of their initial applications for and redeterminations of Medicaid eligibility whether they have other sources of health coverage. In addition, States must independently identify health coverage of Medicaid beneficiaries by matching States' coverage files with those of third parties. States must also conduct diagnosis and trauma edits on Medicaid claims to identify potential casualty and liability coverage.[11]

States' identification systems require continual updates of beneficiary information and potential third-party liability (TPL) information to accurately identify liable third parties. Regular updates allow States to make new matches, but also to update information from previous matches because beneficiary coverage status can change over time.

Third-Party Payment

When States identify probable TPL, they, or a contractor operating on their behalf, use two methods to ensure that Medicaid is the payer of last resort: cost avoidance and pay and chase.

Cost Avoidance. Cost avoidance is the method that States use to avoid payment when other insurance resources are available to the beneficiary. When States recognize claims as belonging to beneficiaries who have other insurance, they will deny payment and return the claims to providers, who are then required to bill and collect payment from any liable third parties. If States have electronic claims processing systems, they can automatically deny payment when claims enter their systems. Federal regulations generally require States to use cost avoidance when probable TPL is established.[12]

Cost avoidance is the most cost-effective way to ensure that Medicaid is the payer of last resort. When States avoid costs, they do not pay money upfront or spend resources on recovery. Once States deny payment and notify providers of a liable third party, providers should bill future claims to the third party first, rather than the States.

Pay and chase. In contrast, the pay-and-chase method occurs when States pay providers for submitted claims and then attempt to recover payments from liable third parties. States may pay and chase claims for two primary reasons: postpayment identification of TPL and Social Security Act exceptions to cost avoidance. First, if States identify probable TPL after payment, Medicaid will have to pay and chase claims. If a third party, such as Medicare, awards retroactive eligibility to a beneficiary, Medicaid will also have to pay and chase claims.[13] Second, the Social Security Act requires that States pay and chase claims instead of using cost avoidance when (1) the service is prenatal care, (2) the service is preventive pediatric care, or (3) coverage is through a parent whose obligation to pay support is enforced by the States' child enforcement agency.[14] However, the President's fiscal year (FY) 2013 budget contained a provision to remove these Social Security Act exceptions to cost avoidance to strengthen TPL.[15]

In general, States obtain recoveries by billing third parties directly and receiving reimbursements from them. For instance, States commonly use this process when trying to obtain recoveries from third-party health insurance.

Some types of third parties require specialized pay-and-chase recovery processes. Specifically, States engage in specialized recovery processes when seeking reimbursements from Medicare and settlements involving either casualty insurance or probated estates.

When seeking reimbursements from Medicare, States may not bill Medicare directly. Instead, they can direct providers to bill Medicare for claims for which States have already paid providers. States must decide whether to take this step and, if so, how they should obtain reimbursement from providers. Some States choose to immediately recover money from providers for Medicare-related claims and do not wait for providers to be reimbursed by Medicare. Some States give providers a defined period (e.g., 60 days) to receive reimbursement from Medicare before they recover money or disallow future payments. These States may not recover money during this period, or afterward, if providers can prove that they did not receive reimbursement from Medicare. Other States do not attempt to recover payments for Medicare-related claims for which they have paid providers.

In casualty insurance and probated estates, States may have to negotiate or wait for a settlement or court decision before they can recover money for billed claims. Casualty recoveries will be limited to the amount of the settlement that is designated for reimbursement of medical costs.[16] States' ability to recover money from probated estates depends on the value of the estates and whether other creditors are also making claims against them.

To obtain pay-and-chase recoveries from absent parents, States enter into cooperative agreements with State-run child support enforcement agencies.[17]

During the pay-and-chase process, States may not recover all amounts billed to third parties for several reasons. States may bill third parties for claims for which they are not liable. This may occur when a service for which Medicaid paid is not covered by the third party or the third party did not cover the beneficiary on the date of service. Alternatively, third parties may be liable for a claim but be uncooperative, refusing to pay or to process a claim. In these cases, the third party may refuse to pay the entire claim or try to pay a lesser amount. States may contest the denial and resubmit the claim to the third party. Finally, States may determine that it is no longer cost-effective to try to recover a reimbursement on a claim. Based on Federal regulations and State Medicaid plans, each State sets a dollar threshold or other guidelines for following up on claims owed to them by liable third parties.[18] Using the threshold or guidelines amount, States determine whether it is cost-effective to devote resources to following up on an unpaid claim.[19]

Hiring TPL Contractors

States may choose to conduct all benefits coordination activities themselves or hire a contractor to conduct some or all of these activities. The range of responsibilities that States delegate to contractors varies. For instance, some States delegate all coordination of benefits to contractors. Other States conduct most coordination of benefits activities themselves but have agreements with contractors to perform certain limited functions.

TPL Reporting

States submit a Quarterly Expense Report (CMS-64) to CMS. The CMS-64 is a statement of expenditures for which States are entitled to Federal reimbursement.[20] The CMS-64 also includes information on recoveries, including TPL-related recoveries.

The CMS-64.9A, an attachment to the CMS-64, describes TPL activity. On the CMS-64.9A, States must report the amounts they avoided paying to third parties and the amounts they recovered from third parties. Some types of third parties, such as Medicare, are specific line items on this attachment. However, not all types of third parties are listed separately.

The CMS-64.9A does not include certain types of information. First, regarding pay and chase, CMS does not require States to report the amount of money they attempted to recover or the amount denied by third parties. Second, regarding cost avoidance, States do not report how they calculated cost avoidance. CMS does not have a standard formula for calculating cost avoidance, and States' methods for calculating it vary. For instance, some States calculate the amount Medicaid avoided paying as the difference between the amount that Medicaid would have paid and the amount that Medicaid actually paid. By contrast, other States report the total amount of a claim as savings, regardless of what Medicaid would have covered.

States submit the CMS-64 and its attachments through the Medicaid Budget and Expenditure System (MBES) and certify that the dollars reported are correct.

CMS uses the reported recovery information, including TPL-related recoveries, to compute the Federal financial participation (FFP) amount for the States' Medicaid program costs. However, CMS does not factor reported cost avoidance into the FFP amount because it does not involve dollars returned to States by third parties.

TPL Provisions of the DRA

The DRA contained provisions that were designed to enhance States' ability to identify and recover payment from liable third parties. The law clarified the list of entities considered third parties by including specific entities that were previously not listed, such as pharmacy benefit managers.[21] In addition, the DRA required that States have laws requiring specified health insurers and certain other third parties to (1) provide States with information on health insurance coverage, (2) accept the State's right of recovery, (3) allow States 3 years after the date of service to submit claims, and (4) not deny or refuse to pay claims for procedural reasons.[22] These provisions took effect on January 1, 2006.[23] According to CMS staff, as of April 2012, all States except Florida and the District of Columbia had the necessary laws in place.

There are some exceptions to the 3-year timely filing rule under the DRA. For instance, when Medicare is the liable third-party payer, fee-for-service providers have only 1 year after the date of service to submit claims under provisions of the Patient Protection and Affordable Care Act (ACA).[24] If Medicare awards a Medicaid beneficiary retroactive eligibility, the 1-year timely filing requirement may be waived.[25] In addition, TRICARE claims filing regulations, issued before enactment of the DRA, also require that claims be submitted no later than 1 year after the date of service.[26]

Related Work

OIG has reported problems with TPL. In 2001, OIG found that Medicaid was at risk of losing over 80 percent of the dollars it paid and chased for pharmacy claims in 32 States.[27] It also found that almost three-quarters of States reported that third parties refused to process or pay pharmacy claims.[28]

GAO has also reported problems with TPL. A 2006 GAO report found that States encountered problems verifying which Medicaid beneficiaries had private insurance and recovering payments from third parties.[29] Not all third parties were willing to provide access to their coverage files, and some third parties imposed barriers to coverage identification. For example, some pharmacy benefit managers ignored or denied States' requests for verification information, citing privacy provisions in the Health Insurance Portability and Accountability Act of 1996 (HIPAA) or claiming that they were not liable parties. Other third parties and contractors would not participate in data-matching agreements.

Fourteen States estimated their combined losses because of problems recovering payments from third parties to be between $184 million and $196 million per year.[30]

METHODOLOGY

To determine trends that influenced State savings from liable third parties, we analyzed data on savings from cost avoidance and pay and chase, and on money at risk of not being recovered. We also surveyed States regarding factors that (1) helped them save money that third parties should pay and (2) made saving money more challenging.

Scope

This study covered all 50 States and the District of Columbia.

The focus was on savings from fee-for-service claims and, to the extent that they are included in States' reports to CMS, managed care claims. Approximately one-third of States included some information from managed care claims in their CMS-64 reports.

We analyzed trends in State savings from 2001 to 2011, the period since the last OIG study. Our assessment of factors that influenced State savings was focused on more recent periods. We realized through extensive conversations with States that collecting data on the factors that influenced State savings for 11 years would be intensely burdensome to them. We also realized that in some cases data were not available. Instead, we collected data on these factors for as much of that time as was reasonable (e.g., pointin-time, or FYs 2010 and 2011). These periods are described in more detail below.

Data Sources and Data Collection

Annual TPL Data. We obtained State-reported CMS-64 and CMS-64.9A data from MBES for each State for FYs 2001 through 2011. We used these data to determine States' total Medicaid expenditures and their savings from, and trends in, cost avoidance and pay-and-chase over the 11-year period. The data collected are totals, reflecting the Federal and State shares.

Data Collection From States. In November 2011, we sent a data collection instrument to each State's TPL coordinator. The instrument had two sections—a data request and a survey. We obtained a 100-percent response rate to the data collection instrument, although some States could not provide portions of the requested data. Where appropriate, item response rates are included below.

We asked States to provide data on their recovery rate for pay-and-chase claims and on the amount of money they believed was owed to them by third parties.[31] We collected these data separately for Medicare, health insurance, casualty insurance, and probated estates. The response rate for items in the data request section of the collection instrument ranged from 88 to 98 percent.

We collected data on States' recovery rates in two ways. First, for Medicare and health insurance, we asked States for the total amount that they billed for FYs 2010 and 2011 and, of that, the total amount collected for each year. We requested these data for only 2 years to reduce the burden on States. Second, for casualty insurance and probated estates, we asked States to report their rate of return for closed cases. We did not specify a time period for the self-reported rates.

We also asked States to provide data on the amount of money that they considered to be at risk of not being recovered. To do so, we asked States to provide their best estimate of money that they believed was owed to them from third parties. To reduce the likelihood that claims still in the process of being paid would be reported as dollars at risk of not being recovered, we instructed States to include only dollars they had considered to be at risk 6 months before the survey was due.

The survey section of the collection instrument focused on factors that might influence States' savings from third parties. We asked States which activities were most useful for identification of third parties. We also asked which factors had improved their ability to avoid costs or recover payments since 2006. Similarly, we asked about challenges related to coordination of benefits activities. Finally, we asked States about their CMS-64 reporting activities, about their use of TPL contractors, and for basic program information. The response rate for items in the survey section ranged from 96 to 100 percent.

Data Analysis

TPL Trends and Total Savings. We analyzed the data that States reported to CMS to identify the percentage change in total savings from cost avoidance and pay and chase between 2001 and 2011, the percentage change in the total amount of money that States expended over these 11 years, and the cumulative amount that States saved over this period.[32] We compared the percentage change in States' savings to the percentage change in total Medicaid expenditures. We then calculated the percentage change in savings related to cost avoidance, pay and chase, probated estates, and subgroups of these categories that States report to CMS. To obtain the cumulative amount in total savings, we summed all States' cost avoidance and pay-and-chase savings for all 11 years.

We analyzed differences among States; however, this information is not included in this report. While we found differences among States, we did not have contextual data on State demographics and other factors. Without this contextual information, our analysis of State comparisons was largely inconclusive.

Rates of Recovery. We calculated recovery rates both for Medicare and for health insurance pay-and-chase claims. To calculate the recovery rate for Medicare, we divided the amount of money each State collected from Medicare in 2011 by the total amount that State billed to Medicare for pay-and-chase claims. We also performed this calculation for health insurance recoveries.

Money at Risk of Not Being Collected. To calculate the money at risk of not being collected, we added up the money that States reported for Medicare, health insurance, casualty insurance, and probated estates. For Medicare and health insurance, we reported the dollars at risk exactly as States reported them. For casualty insurance and probated estates, we adjusted the amounts that States reported to provide a more accurate account of the money that States are likely to recover.[33]

Factors That Influence State Savings. We analyzed States' responses to survey questions about factors that influenced savings to determine those that were most influential. We also reviewed States' open-ended responses to provide context for factors that States identified as "very challenging."

Limitations

All data are State reported. We did not independently verify the accuracy of data that States reported to CMS or to OIG.

Some portion of cost-avoided dollars cannot, by definition, be quantified. For example, States cannot identify savings from cost avoidance that occurs when a provider correctly submits a claim for reimbursement to a third party rather than to Medicaid.

States' calculations of cost avoidance may be affected by variations in tracking methods. For example, some States track the entire amount that was billed for a cost-avoided claim as savings, while others track only the amount that Medicaid would have paid for that claim as savings. However, these data are sufficient to represent broad trends in savings over time. It is likely that States reported data in the same way in 2011 as in 2001.

Standards

This study was conducted in accordance with the *Quality Standards for Inspection and Evaluation* issued by the Council of the Inspectors General on Integrity and Efficiency.

FINDINGS

Medicaid TPL Savings Increased, but 44 States Reported $4 Billion Is at Risk of Not Being Recovered

Overall, States reported increased savings from both cost avoidance and pay and chase between 2001 and 2011. Specifically, savings increased from nearly $34 billion in 2001 to slightly more than $72 billion in 2011, representing a 114-percent increase. However, because States generally were not able to recover all of the money they went after, a significant amount remains at risk of not being recovered. Cumulatively, 44 States reported $4 billion is at risk.[34]

States' reported growth in cost-avoidance and pay-and-chase savings does not appear to be tied to growth in Medicaid expenditures or in the percentage of Medicaid beneficiaries with another source of insurance. For example, reported expenditures increased 47 percent from 2001 to 2011, compared to TPL's 114-percent growth. Such growth suggests that TPL savings outpaced growth in Medicaid expenditures. Further, the percentage of beneficiaries with another source of health insurance generally remained stable between 2002 and 2010.[35]

States' Reported Savings from Cost Avoidance Drove Growth in TPL Savings

States' reported cost-avoidance savings accounted for most TPL growth and total savings between 2001 and 2011. States' reported savings from cost avoidance grew 117 percent, from $33 billion to $70 billion, between 2001 and 2011. Cumulatively, States reported that they avoided paying $512 billion from 2001 to 2011. Had States paid for these services, reported Medicaid expenditures could have been 13 percent greater. See Chart 1 for TPL savings trends from 2001–2011 by cost avoidance, pay and chase, and probated estates.

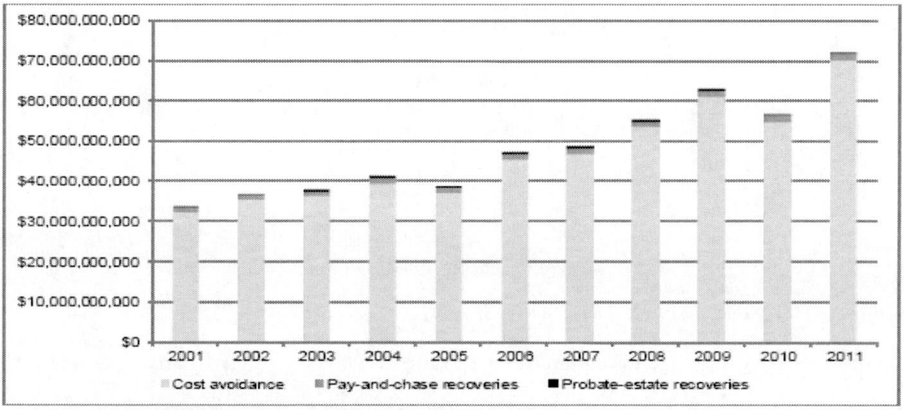

Source: OIG analysis of CMS-64.9A reports, 2012.

Chart 1. TPL Savings From 2001 to 2011.

Although similar proportions of Medicaid beneficiaries have Medicare or health insurance as third-party payers nationally, Medicare makes up about 80 percent of total costs avoided. A variety of factors contributes to this, including that cost avoidance is generally easier for Medicare claims than for other types of third parties. Because Medicare beneficiaries tend to keep Medicare after they become eligible, once States have third-party coverage information they can avoid payment for all future claims. In contrast, other forms of third-party coverage, such as health insurance obtained through an employer, are more likely to fluctuate and result in multiple updates to State systems.

Although Medicare traditionally has been the largest driver of cost avoidance since 2001, States reported some recent gains in cost avoidance from third-party health insurance. For example, in 2001, health insurance made up 10 percent of total costs avoided; by 2011, it had grown to 18 percent. These gains suggest that the DRA had some effect on States' ability to avoid costs, likely through improvements in States' identification of third parties. See Chart 2 for more detail.

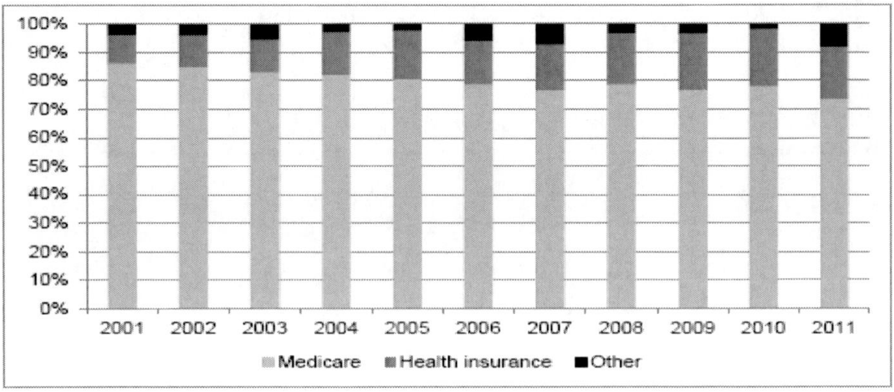

Source: OIG analysis of CMS-64.9A reports, 2012.

Chart 2. Cost-Avoidance Percentages Over Time, by Type of Third-Party Insurance.

Increases in State Recoveries Also Contributed to TPL Savings

Although State recoveries through pay and chase make up only about 3 percent of total TPL savings, these recoveries are increasing. States' pay-and-chase recoveries from health insurance, Medicare, casualty settlements, and cooperative agreements increased by 61 percent, from $1 billion to $1.6 billion, between 2001 and 2011. Cumulative pay-and-chase recoveries over this period resulted in $14.7 billion in savings for States.

As with cost avoidance, the proportion of pay-and-chase recoveries varies by type of third-party. Specifically, pay-and-chase recoveries from health insurance accounted for 50 percent of cumulative pay-and-chase recoveries between 2001 and 2011, while Medicare accounted for 18 percent of such recoveries. See Chart 3 for more detail.

Moreover, the percentage of recoveries from health insurance is growing. In 2001, health insurance accounted for 42 percent of recoveries from pay and chase, compared to 62 percent of total dollars recovered in 2011. Similar to cost avoidance, these gains suggest that the DRA had some effect on States' ability to recover money, possibly because of an increased ability to identify claims that need to be recovered or to the DRA's expansion of the timely filing limit to 3 years.

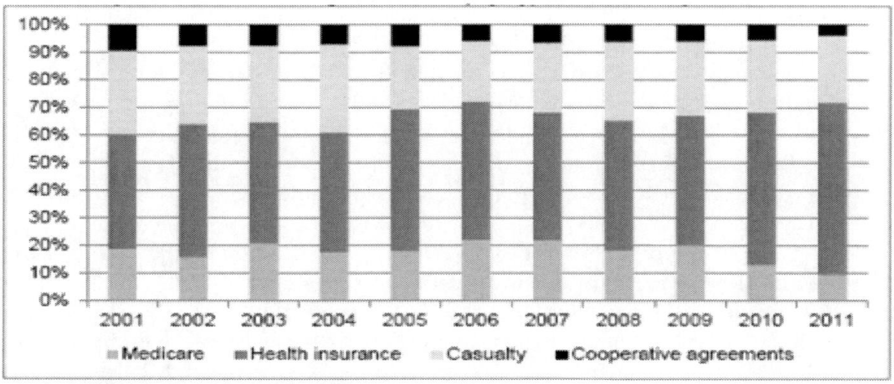

Source: OIG analysis of CMS-64.9A reports, 2012.

Note: Casualty insurance and cooperative agreements are other sources through which States may recover funds from third parties. Casualty coverage may be a source of TPL if Medicaid paid for medical expenses resulting from accidental injury that should have been covered by casualty insurance. Cooperative agreements assist States in pursuing a liable third party, for example, to identify parents who are obligated to pay for the health care of Medicaid recipients.

Chart 3. Pay-and-Chase Percentages Over Time, by Type of Third-Party Insurance

Table 1. Dollars at Risk of Not Being Recovered

Type	Dollars at Risk	Percentage of Dollars at Risk
Health insurance	$2,356,853,103	57%
Probated estates*	$931,268,692	22%
Casualty*	$744,684,814	18%
Medicare	$110,868,962	3%
Total	$4,143,675,571	100%

*The dollars for probated estates and casualty reflect the average amount States expect to recover and consider to be owed to them, not the entire amount of the probated estate or casualty claim. Source: OIG analysis of data collection instrument responses, 2012.

Despite Increased Savings, States Reported Potential Recoveries at Risk

As of June 30, 2011, 44 States cumulatively reported $4.1 billion that they believe is owed by third parties and is at risk of not being recovered.[36] This sum includes Federal and State dollars. The term "dollars at risk" refers only to claims that States pay and chase; cost-avoided dollars are never at risk because they are never expended by States. Table 1 shows the money that States report being owed by third parties.

The disparity between the amount that States tried to recover from third-party health insurance and the amount actually collected may contribute to high amounts of dollars at risk. On average, 45 States reported recovering 18 percent of what they billed to third-party health insurance in 2011. These low recovery rates may be due in part to States' challenges to reimbursement, which are discussed in more detail later in the report.

States experience higher recovery rates from Medicare than from third-party health insurance, contributing to fewer dollars at risk. The average recovery rate in 2011 for Medicare was 69 percent among the 32 States that were able to provide data. It is unclear why Medicare recovery rates are higher, but one explanation could be that some States automatically recover money from providers when Medicare is the third party. By contrast, when a health insurance carrier is the third party, States generally submit bills directly to the carrier and must wait for its response.

States Reported That Improvements to Their Processes Facilitated TPL Savings, But Challenges Remain

States identified several factors that facilitated improvements in cost avoidance and pay and chase, despite also reporting some longstanding challenges. In general, process improvements, such as information technology and use of contractors, facilitated these improvements, which led to greater savings. At the same time, States reported continued challenges with third parties when trying to identify insurance coverage and recover payments similar to those identified by States in previous OIG and GAO studies. In addition, States reported challenges—caused, they say, by laws and regulations—that hinder the recovery of payments.

States Reported That Their Use of Electronic Systems and Contractors Facilitated Improved Savings

Forty-Five States Reported That Their Electronic Systems Facilitated Improvements in Their Identification, Cost Avoidance, and Recovery Efforts.

States indicated that electronic systems improved the efficiency with which they were able to identify beneficiaries with third-party insurance. This improved efficiency resulted from: (1) conducting online verification of coverage and (2) having electronic data-matching agreements with third parties. Forty-two States reported that at least one of these systems was "very useful" for identifying third parties. See Table 2 for a breakdown of the number of States that reported that each system was very useful for identifying third parties.

Table 2. Electronic Systems That States Reported as Very Useful for Identifying Third Parties

Electronic System	Reported as Very Useful	Percentage of States
Online verification	37	73%
Via third-party Web site	36	71%
Via TPL clearinghouse vendor	20	39%
Having electronic data matching agreements with third parties	34	68%

Source: OIG analysis of State data collection instrument responses, 2012.

Electronic systems helped States identify third parties more efficiently, which helped States save money. For instance, verifying coverage online through a third-party Web site is quicker than phoning or faxing a third party. In addition, States reported that using TPL clearinghouses—vendors with electronic agreements with many insurance companies—was helpful. States pay clearinghouses to match coverage information for beneficiaries against a clearinghouse's collection of data. Lastly, data-matching agreements increase efficiency because they allow States to check for third-party insurance for many beneficiaries at one time. In these cases, States share their Medicaid enrollment with third parties, which then compare States' lists to their covered individuals and produce a report of all matches for States.

Similarly, using electronic systems increased States' efficiency in avoiding costs and recovering payments. Thirty-six States reported that increases in electronic claims or electronic billing significantly improved their ability to save money. Electronic claims occur when providers submit claims electronically for services provided to Medicaid beneficiaries to States for payment. Electronic billing occurs when States send their invoices for reimbursement to third parties via electronic means. Both of these systems may help States save money because automated processes replace manual processes. For example, because electronic claims from providers are transmitted directly to States' claim management processing systems, claim reviews, TPL checks, and cost-avoidance activities happen automatically, rather than manually.

In addition, States' ability to receive payments electronically from third parties appears to have had some positive effect on savings. As of December 2011, 32 States reported accepting electronic payments. These States demonstrated a 78-percent increase in recoveries between 2001 and 2011. On the other hand, the 18 States that did not accept electronic payments had an 18-percent increase in recoveries over the same period.

States Reported That Assistance from Contractors Facilitated Improvements in Their Identification and Recovery Efforts

Forty-seven States used a contractor for at least one TPL activity, and all but two of these States indicated that contractor assistance was either useful for identifying third parties or improved States' ability to collect pay-and-chase claims.

States reported that the most helpful functions contractors provide are identification and verification. Overall, 29 States that have contractors indicated that such assistance was very useful in identifying third-party insurance. States indicated that contractors' data-matching agreements with out-of-state third parties helped them identify third-party insurance. Because contractors were more likely to have relationships with a wider array of third parties, they could more easily develop data-matching agreements than States could.

States reported that the second-most helpful contractor-assisted function was conducting collections. Overall, 27 States that used contractors indicated that such collection assistance with pay-and-chase claims from third parties significantly improved States' ability to recover money. For example, some States indicated that contractors may be useful in doing followup work on claims that are hard to recover.

States Reported Longstanding Challenges with Third Parties When Trying to Identify Insurance Coverage and Recover Payments

Although States' TPL savings improved, they continue to face challenges in maximizing savings from third parties. States reported challenges in identifying third parties and recovering payments through pay and chase. In fact, 49 States identified at least one part of these activities as "very challenging." However, data are inconclusive as to whether States that identified more challenges than others have less in TPL savings.

In passing the DRA, Congress attempted to mitigate challenges in identifying third parties and recovering payments.[37] However, we found that many of the challenges that States reported are similar to those reported in 2001 and 2006.[38, 39]

States Continue To Face Challenges Identifying Beneficiaries With Third-Party Insurance Because Third Parties Do Not Always Provide Complete Coverage Information. All States reported that identifying third parties was challenging. Identification of third-party insurance is the first, and key, step in saving money through TPL. Without the appropriate information, States cannot avoid costs or recover payments.

Although the details may have changed for certain challenges, identification has historically been challenging for States. In 2001, States reported concerns about inaccurate or incomplete information in coverage files and difficulty identifying claims processing entities.[40] In 2006, States noted problems with third parties' ignoring their requests for coverage information and being unwilling to share data electronically.[41] In 2011, States reported challenges with third parties' submitting explanation of benefit (EOB) forms that were confusing or incomplete. See Table 3 for a complete list of challenges related to identification of third parties that States identified in 2011.[42]

Table 3. Challenges That States Reported Related to Identification

Specific Challenge With Identification	Percentage of States That Reported the Challenge in 2011
Third-party concerns about HIPAA and releasing insurance coverage information to States	90%
EOB forms from third parties that are confusing or incomplete	86%
Cooperation from pharmacy benefit managers	84%
Obtaining data about beneficiaries' third-party insurance from State or Federal entities	78%
Obtaining data from TRICARE on Medicaid beneficiaries with potential TRICARE coverage	74%

Source: OIG analysis of State data collection instrument responses, 2012.

The most frequently cited challenge to identification was third-party concern about HIPAA and whether third parties can release information to

States. States are exempt from HIPAA under the privacy rule's exception for the use and disclosure of protected health information for treatment, payment, and health care operations.[43] CMS has also issued guidance on this issue.[44] However, States indicated that third parties continue to use HIPAA as an excuse to not provide information. For example, one State reported:

> Many commercial carriers frequently quote HIPAA and then refuse to verify coverage when our State agency contacts them. We frequently must go through their compliance office in an attempt to get clearance. Once we obtain clearance it does not always help us the next time we need to verify coverage. Carriers feel it is a violation of HIPAA to confirm the existence of coverage and the lives covered.

The next most frequently cited challenge to identification was that EOB forms States receive from third parties are either difficult to interpret or incomplete. Inaccurate and incomplete information on EOB forms hinders States' attempts to determine whether they correctly identified the liable third party. When a third party refuses liability, it denies the claim via an EOB form. The EOB form should indicate the reason for denying a claim (i.e., that the third party refuses its coverage liability). However, there is no standard format for the EOB form. States indicated that, even across national plans, EOB forms are inconsistent and that data may not be easily identifiable or be in the same spot on the form. This is problematic for States because "it can be very difficult ... to understand them and key it correctly." In addition, States reported that third parties did not always submit all information on the EOB form denying States' requests for payment. One State provided this example: "There are some companies that do not provide a complete EOB the first time around. Claims are corrected and resubmitted based on the first EOB, only to receive a second EOB with new items that need to be resolved."

Another challenge that States reported was lack of cooperation from pharmacy benefit managers. States have reported this challenge since 2001. In fact, in 2001, OIG found that more States had problems with pharmacy benefit managers than with all other third parties combined.[45] The DRA attempted to increase cooperation from pharmacy benefit managers by clarifying that they are third parties, and as such must accept States' right of recovery. CMS has also issued guidance to this effect.[46] Yet in 2011, States again reported that pharmacy benefit managers were uncooperative. One State provided this example: "They make you guess a date [of coverage eligibility] and then will tell you yes or no." States indicated that pharmacy benefit managers will not provide eligibility dates for covered beneficiaries, will not verify coverage unless a State has the policy number, and may be unwilling to speak to States' representatives.

Finally, States reported challenges obtaining data about third-party coverage from State and Federal entities. Some States cited problems getting workers' compensation or child support claims needed to identify additional sources of third-party insurance. States also reported that some entities cite Internal Revenue Service or Social Security Administration security requirements that prevent them from disclosing Social Security numbers and other personal identifiers required for data matching. In addition, States reported that TRICARE is challenging, mostly because it will conduct only one data match per year with each State.

States Continue To Face Challenges Recovering Payments Because Third Parties Refuse To Process or Pay Claims. All but one State reported continuing challenges with third parties refusing to process or pay claims, despite State laws requiring third-party cooperation that were enacted pursuant to the DRA. Generally, States have reported these challenges since 2001. In 2001, States reported that claims were not processed or were returned with vague denial codes, and that some pharmacy benefit managers would not process claims because their clients had not authorized them to do so.[47] In 2006, States reported that third parties refused to respond to or cooperate on claims filed for payment by States.[48] In 2011, States reported similar challenges, such as third parties' issuing denials for procedural reasons. See Table 4 for a complete list of the challenges related to third-party refusal to pay or process claims, whether States reported the challenges in the past, and whether the DRA sought to address them.[49]

The most frequently cited longstanding challenge to recovering payments is denial from third parties for procedural reasons or with no explanation. In 2011, 42 States reported that $3.4 billion of the $7 billion that they billed to third-party health insurance was denied. Although third parties may legitimately deny claims (e.g., if the insurer did not cover the Medicaid beneficiary), denials for procedural reasons or with no explanation are not considered legitimate. In fact, the DRA specifically required States to pass laws prohibiting third parties from refusing to reimburse States for procedural reasons. It is unclear what portion of the $3.4 billion in denied claims was inappropriately denied by third parties and still eligible for collection. However, some portion of that money may contribute to the amount that States reported as at risk.

Table 4. Challenges States Reported About Third-Party Refusal to Process or Pay Claims

Challenge	Identified in 2001 OIG Report	Identified in 2006 GAO Report	DRA Attempted To Address	Identified in 2011 (This Study)	Percentage of States That Reported Challenge in 2011
Denial by third parties	X			X	98%
For procedural reasons	X	X	X	X	96%
No explanation	X			X	88%
Third parties not responding when State submits bills	X	X	X	X	92%
Third parties not abiding by 3-year timely filing rules				X	88%
Third-party documentation submitted with reimbursement does not indicate which claims are being reimbursed				X	88%
Third parties not accepting States' right to collect	X	X	X	X	82%
Pharmacy benefit managers claim they do not have the authority to reimburse States directly	X	X	X	X	82%

Source: OIG analysis of State data collection instrument responses, 2012.

An additional longstanding reported challenge is third parties' failing to respond to States' claims. For instance, in 2011, 41 States reported that third parties did not respond to $2 billion of the $7 billion billed to third-party health insurance. When this happens, States may lose money.

Another challenge that States have reported since 2001 is that third parties do not accept States' right to collect reimbursements. One State indicated that this was a particular problem with out-of-State third-party insurers. Another

State indicated that there still appeared to be some confusion about Medicaid being the payer of last resort.

A final challenge States have reported since 2001 is that pharmacy benefit managers claim they do not have the authority to reimburse States directly.

Despite State laws requiring third-party cooperation that were enacted pursuant to the DRA, in 2011, half of States reported this issue as "very challenging." Several States reported that pharmacy benefit managers claim they can reimburse States only when beneficiaries' employers have authorized them to do so. In refusing to reimburse States, pharmacy benefit managers have contended that the Employee Retirement Income Security Act of 1974 (ERISA) prevents reimbursement to States by pharmacy benefit managers for employer-governed health benefit plans.[50] Pharmacy benefit managers have also argued that they must refuse reimbursement to States according to procedural restrictions chosen by plan sponsors.[51] These arguments have proved unsuccessful for pharmacy benefit managers in recent litigation.[52]

States Reported That Certain Laws and Regulations Created Challenges to Recovering Payments

In addition to longstanding challenges from third parties, all States reported that particular laws and regulations, or the lack thereof, are challenging to recovery efforts. Specifically, the Medicare and TRICARE 1-year timely filing limits were most frequently reported to be "very challenging." See Table 5 for a list of specific challenges related to current laws and regulations.[53]

Table 5. Challenges That States Reported With Current Laws and Regulations

Challenge	Percentage of States That Reported Challenge in 2011
Medicare 1-year timely filing limit	98%
TRICARE 1-year timely filing limit	92%
Lack of enforceable penalties for third parties that refuse to reimburse States	90%
Inability to bill Medicare directly	88%
Lack of rules requiring third parties to reimburse in a timely manner	82%

Source: OIG analysis of State data collection instrument responses, 2012.

Medicare Timely Filing Limit Is Challenging. States reported that the Medicare 1-year timely filing limit creates barriers to recovery. Because States cannot bill Medicare directly, they must decide whether and how to recover money from providers. Some States direct providers to first bill Medicare and then forward payment to States once it is received. If States do not discover the third-party insurance in time for providers to meet the 1-year timely filing deadline, States lose that money. Some States may not attempt to recover Medicare claims because it is not cost effective.

States may remedy the problem by recovering money from providers, regardless of whether providers are paid by Medicare. In this case, States recover their payments, but providers may not complete their recovery from Medicare in time to get paid. However, States expressed concern about the consequences of taking money back from providers when they do not expect the providers to recover the money from Medicare. Multiple States indicated that providers may choose not to participate in Medicaid because of this challenge and are concerned that this may limit beneficiary access. Some States are so concerned that they do not attempt to recover money from providers for Medicare claims.

Medicare regulations allow providers an exception to the 1-year timely filing limit, but States expressed concern that the exception is of limited use to providers in getting their money back.[54] If CMS, or one of its contractors, determines that beneficiaries were retroactively awarded Medicare coverage and States have recovered their money from providers, providers will be granted additional time to file claims with Medicare. However, States reported that the requirements for meeting the conditions for exception to the timely filing limit are challenging. At the time of our data collection, providers had to produce the letter notifying the beneficiary of retroactive Medicare entitlement to qualify for the exception. States reported that providers often do not have, and cannot get, this letter. CMS changed this requirement after we completed our data collection. As of August 27, 2012, if providers do not have access to this letter, Medicare contractors can use Medicare databases to verify retroactive eligibility.[55]

TRICARE's 1-Year Timely Filing Limit Is Challenging. States reported that TRICARE's 1-year timely filing limit is also challenging, primarily because TRICARE allows each State one data match per year. States may find claims that were already paid and potentially should have been paid by TRICARE, but are for dates of service more than 1 year previous and are past the 1-year window.

The high percentage of States reporting that TRICARE's 1-year timely filing limit is challenging may be due to lack of clarity about TRICARE's policy. Specifically, States may have a different interpretation of the start date of the 1-year window, depending on which source of TRICARE guidance they consult. TRICARE regulations indicate that States have 1 year from the date of service to file a claim.[56] The *TRICARE Reimbursement Manual* extends that window by allowing States 1 year from the date of the annual data match. According to the *TRICARE Reimbursement Manual*, States may file claims no later than 1 year after the: (1) date of service, (2) date the prescription was filled, (3) date of discharge if the services were rendered during an inpatient admission, or (4) the date a State received the results of the annual data match.[57] However, the sample billing agreement that States sign to claim reimbursement from TRICARE does not mention the four options and indicates only that claims must be filed "no later than one year following the date of service or the date of discharge for inpatient services."[58] Although the billing agreement indicates that TRICARE contractors can grant waivers to the claims filing deadline, the requirements for obtaining a waiver are not listed.

Some States and CMS staff have indicated that they were not aware of alternatives to using the date of service for the start of the 1-year timely filing deadline.

States Lack an Enforcement Mechanism for Uncooperative Third Parties. States indicated that the lack of penalties for refusal to reimburse and lack of rules for timely reimbursement were challenges to achieving TPL savings. Without a mechanism to enforce penalties, States have no influence over third parties and few resources to compel payment.

Although States' Attorneys General may seek legal action against third parties, States indicated that these efforts are resource intensive and the outcomes are uncertain and may not be cost effective. In addition, there are no rules for how long third parties have to reimburse States once States have submitted a bill. Lacking rules requiring third parties to reimburse States in a timely manner, States bill third parties multiple times and have outstanding balances in their fiscal systems for indefinite periods.

CONCLUSION AND RECOMMENDATIONS

Since 2001, States have made sizable gains in TPL savings. Improvements in States' processes and changes enacted by the DRA appear to have had a positive effect. However, States reported that $4 billion remains at risk of not being recovered, so further efforts to improve TPL savings are warranted.

Longstanding challenges persist in recovering payments from third parties. In particular, States reported challenges in getting third parties to provide complete insurance coverage information and to process or pay claims. States have been reporting these challenges since 2001. States also indicated that challenges involving current laws and regulations limited their ability to recover payments.

Based on the amount of money at risk of not being recovered and the longstanding challenges that States continue to face, we make three recommendations to CMS to strengthen Medicaid TPL outcomes.

CMS should:

Work With States To Address Longstanding Challenges Working With Third Parties To Identify Insurance Coverage and Recover Payments.

CMS should work with States, and potentially with third parties, to address challenges related to identification and recovery of payments. Because States face similar TPL challenges, CMS could help coordinate their efforts. In addition, many of the third parties have coverage across the country, so a broad plan, rather than individual State negotiations, would be appropriate.

At a minimum, CMS should address the challenges with identifying third parties and recovering payments that were identified in this report. This could include collecting and disseminating examples of State best practices for working with third parties or methods to educate third parties on particular topics (e.g., HIPAA, obligation to respond to States, or not denying claims with no explanation).

CMS could also explore ways to take an active role in facilitating States' coordination of benefits activities. This could include (1) acting as a liaison for data-sharing agreements, (2) coordinating with TRICARE, and (3) working with States to determine whether CMS has a role to play in working with third parties that are consistently uncooperative across a number of States.

CMS's actions to address State challenges should pay particular attention to pharmacy benefit managers. Since OIG's 2001 study, States have consistently reported that pharmacy benefit managers are uncooperative. CMS could facilitate efforts to better understand and mitigate pharmacy benefit managers' concerns.

CMS could use the TPL Technical Assistance Group (TAG) to develop solutions to address States' challenges. Or, it could create a task force that includes States and third parties, including key pharmacy benefit managers, to work toward feasible solutions.

Address States' Challenges With 1-Year Timely Filing Limits for Medicare and TRICARE.

Medicare's and TRICARE's filing limits were the two items that had the most "very challenging" responses from States. States may be unable to bill for and recover claims within the 1-year limit, resulting in losses for the States.

To address the Medicare concerns, CMS should ensure that States and providers are aware of and understand the August 2012 change to the policy for requesting an exception to the 1-year timely filing limit for retroactive Medicare eligibility. CMS could issue a State Medicaid Director Letter explaining this change.

To address the TRICARE concerns, CMS could engage in conversations with TRICARE to clarify the policies for the 1-year timely filing limit. CMS could clarify the start date of the timely filing limit. CMS could also ask TRICARE to clarify how its claims processing contractors apply the *TRICARE Reimbursement Manual*'s start date policies when reviewing claims submitted by State Medicaid agencies. They could also discuss the procedures and circumstances, if any, under which States should request waivers. CMS and TRICARE could also discuss whether any changes should be made to the State Agency Billing Agreement to further incorporate the *Reimbursement Manual* guidelines. CMS could then issue guidance to States on TRICARE policies and procedures.

Work To Strengthen Enforcement Mechanisms Designed To Deal With Uncooperative Third Parties.

The DRA enacted solutions for many of the challenges that OIG and GAO found related to working with third parties to identify insurance coverage and recover payments, but States reported that working with third parties remains challenging. The law does not include any enforcement authority to penalize third parties for violations. Enforcement mechanisms would allow States and the Federal Government to send a strong message that third parties must comply with the law, and ultimately help States and the Federal Government recover some of the $4 billion that States report as being at risk.

Enforcement could take many forms. For example, penalties could be assessed if third parties are uncooperative when States attempt to identify or verify coverage. On the recovery end, enforcement could include interest, or a fine, for claims that are not responded to in a given period.

Because different organizations govern different aspects of health insurance, CMS should work with the appropriate Federal and State entities to determine whether these suggestions are feasible enforcement options or whether others exist. For example, to explore possibilities for enforcement related to employer-sponsored health plans subject to ERISA, CMS could work with the Department of Labor. The appropriate divisions within CMS could explore enforcement options for pharmacy benefit managers that contract to provide Medicare services. CMS should also work with States to explore options to strengthen State enforcement mechanisms under State laws and regulations governing insurance. Finally, CMS could consider whether additional congressional action would be helpful.

AGENCY COMMENTS AND OFFICE OF INSPECTOR GENERAL RESPONSE

CMS concurred with our recommendations. For the first recommendation, CMS stated that it will work with States and third parties to address the problems with identifying insurance coverage and recovering payments that are identified in this report. CMS will consult with its TPL TAG to identify what guidance is needed from CMS and will work with States to identify best practices. For the second recommendation, CMS indicated that it would inform States and Medicare providers about the recent change in Medicare's requirements for an exception to the Medicare 1-year timely filing limit. CMS also stated that it would talk with the Department of Defense and States to understand and to clarify policies for the TRICARE 1-year timely filing limit. For the third recommendation, CMS indicated that it would work with States to explore options to strengthen enforcement mechanisms under State laws. CMS also stated that it would review its own existing enforcement authorities. OIG encourages CMS to think broadly about this third recommendation, as we believe that CMS can play a role in facilitating the conversation about additional enforcement authority.

CMS noted that OIG did not adjust States' estimates of dollars at risk for Medicare or health insurance and therefore the overall dollars at risk may be less than reported. CMS asserted that States usually submit claims to health insurance carriers for more than the amount that the carrier is legally liable to pay. OIG acknowledges that actual health insurance liability may reduce the dollars at risk that States are legally entitled to recover from health insurers. However, no reliable estimate of how often States bill above the health insurers' liability cap or the rate of liability reduction is available. Further, OIG does not think it is instructive to look to the average rate of return of 18 percent on health insurance as a proxy measure for reduced liability. The average rate of return reflects reduced liability along with a variety of other factors, chiefly the challenges identified in this report, including payment denials for procedural reasons and nonresponsive third parties.

APPENDIX A. CHALLENGES BY STATE

Table A-1. Challenges That States Reported to Identification and Verification, by State

	Third-party concerns about the Health Insurance Portability and Accountability Act of 1996 and releasing insurance coverage information to States		Confusing or incomplete Explanation of Benefit forms from third parties		Cooperation from pharmacy benefit managers		Obtaining data from State or Federal entities that may have data about beneficiaries' third-party insurance		Obtaining data from TRICARE on Medicaid beneficiaries with potential TRICARE coverage	
State	Very Challenging	Somewhat Challenging	Very Challenging	Somewhat Challenging	Very Challenging	Somewhat Challenging	Very Challenging	Somewhat Challenging	Very Challenging	Somewhat Challenging
Alabama		X		X		X	X			X
Alaska		X				X				
Arizona		X				X	X		X	
Arkansas		X		X		X		X		X
California					X					
Colorado		X		X		X	X			X
Connecticut		X		X				X		
Delaware		X		X		X			X	
District of Columbia										X
Florida		X				X	X			X
Georgia		X		X		X		X		X
Hawaii		X		X		X		X		X
Idaho		X		X		X	X			X
Illinois		X		X		X				

Table A-1. (Continued)

State	Third-party concerns about the Health Insurance Portability and Accountability Act of 1996 and releasing insurance coverage information to States		Confusing or incomplete Explanation of Benefit forms from third parties		Cooperation from pharmacy benefit managers		Obtaining data from State or Federal entities that may have data about beneficiaries' third-party insurance		Obtaining data from TRICARE on Medicaid beneficiaries with potential TRICARE coverage	
	Very Challenging	Somewhat Challenging	Very Challenging	Somewhat Challenging	Very Challenging	Somewhat Challenging	Very Challenging	Somewhat Challenging	Very Challenging	Somewhat Challenging
Indiana				X			X			X
Iowa				X		X	X			
Kansas	X			X		X		X		X
Kentucky		X		X		X	X			X
Louisiana		X	X				X			X
Maine		X		X		X		X		X
Maryland		X	X							X
Massachusetts		X	X			X		X		X
Michigan	X		X		X		X			X
Minnesota	X			X	X			X		
Mississippi		X		X		X		X		X
Missouri		X	X			X		X		X
Montana		X	X			X				X
Nebraska		X		X		X		X		X
Nevada		X		X		X	X			X
New Hampshire		X	X			X				
New Jersey		X		X		X	X			X
New Mexico		X				X				X

	Third-party concerns about the Health Insurance Portability and Accountability Act of 1996 and releasing insurance coverage information to States		Confusing or incomplete Explanation of Benefit forms from third parties		Cooperation from pharmacy benefit managers		Obtaining data from State or Federal entities that may have data about beneficiaries' third-party insurance		Obtaining data from TRICARE on Medicaid beneficiaries with potential TRICARE coverage	
State	Very Challenging	Somewhat Challenging	Very Challenging	Somewhat Challenging	Very Challenging	Somewhat Challenging	Very Challenging	Somewhat Challenging	Very Challenging	Somewhat Challenging
New York		X		X		X	X			X
North Carolina		X		X		X	X			X
North Dakota		X		X		X	X		X	
Ohio	X			X						
Oklahoma	X			X	X		X		X	
Oregon	X			X	X			X		X
Pennsylvania	X		X					X		
Rhode Island		X		X				X		X
South Carolina		X			X		X			
South Dakota	X		X		X		X			
Tennessee		X		X		X	X			
Texas	X			X		X		X	X	
Utah		X		X		X		X		X
Vermont		X		X		X		X		
Virginia		X		X		X	X			X
Washington		X		X	X					
West Virginia	X			X		X		X		X
Wisconsin			X			X		X		X
Wyoming	X		X		X			X		X

Source: Office of Inspector General (OIG) analysis of State data collection instrument responses, 2012.

Table A-2. Challenges That States Reported With Third-Party Refusal To Process or Pay Claims, by State

State	Denials from third parties for procedural reasons		Denials from third parties with no explanation		Third parties not responding when State submits bills		Third parties not abiding by 3-year timely filing rules		Third-party documentation submitted with reimbursement does not indicate which claims are being reimbursed		Third parties not accepting States' right to collect		Pharmacy benefit managers claim they do not have the authority to reimburse States directly	
	Very Challenging	Somewhat Challenging	Very Challenging	Somewhat Challenging	Very Challenging	Somewhat Challenging	Very Challenging	Somewhat Challenging	Very Challenging	Somewhat Challenging	Very Challenging	Somewhat Challenging	Very Challenging	Somewhat Challenging
Alabama	X			X	X			X	X			X	X	
Alaska		X	X			X	X		X			X		
Arizona		X		X						X			X	
Arkansas		X		X		X	X			X		X		X
California		X		X		X		X				X		X
Colorado		X		X		X		X		X		X	X	
Connecticut		X		X		X		X		X		X		X
Delaware		X		X		X		X		X		X	X	
District of Columbia		X		X		X		X		X				X
Florida		X		X		X		X		X		X	X	
Georgia		X		X		X		X		X		X		X
Hawaii		X		X	X			X		X		X		X
Idaho		X		X		X		X		X		X	X	
Illinois		X				X		X		X				X
Indiana		X		X		X		X		X			X	
Iowa		X		X		X		X		X		X	X	

State	Denials from third parties for procedural reasons		Denials from third parties with no explanation		Third parties not responding when State submits bills		Third parties not abiding by 3-year timely filing rules		Third-party documentation submitted with reimbursement does not indicate which claims are being reimbursed		Third parties not accepting States' right to collect		Pharmacy benefit managers claim they do not have the authority to reimburse States directly	
	Very Challenging	Somewhat Challenging	Very Challenging	Somewhat Challenging	Very Challenging	Somewhat Challenging	Very Challenging	Somewhat Challenging	Very Challenging	Somewhat Challenging	Very Challenging	Somewhat Challenging	Very Challenging	Somewhat Challenging
Kansas		X		X		X		X		X		X	X	
Kentucky		X		X		X		X		X		X	X	
Louisiana		X		X		X		X		X		X		X
Maine		X		X		X		X		X		X	X	
Maryland										X				
Massachusetts				X		X		X				X		X
Michigan		X		X		X		X		X		X		
Minnesota		X		X		X		X		X		X		X
Mississippi	X		X		X		X		X		X		X	
Missouri		X		X		X		X		X		X	X	
Montana		X		X	X			X		X		X		
Nebraska		X		X		X			X			X		
Nevada		X		X		X		X		X		X	X	
New Hampshire	X					X		X		X		X	X	
New Jersey		X		X		X		X		X		X	X	
New Mexico		X		X				X		X				X
New York		X		X		X		X		X		X	X	
North Carolina		X		X		X		X		X		X	X	
North Dakota		X		X		X		X		X		X		X
Ohio		X												

Table A-2. (Continued)

State	Denials from third parties for procedural reasons		Denials from third parties with no explanation		Third parties not responding when State submits bills		Third parties not abiding by 3-year timely filing rules		Third-party documentation submitted with reimbursement does not indicate which claims are being reimbursed		Third parties not accepting States' right to collect		Pharmacy benefit managers claim they do not have the authority to reimburse States directly	
	Very Challenging	Somewhat Challenging	Very Challenging	Somewhat Challenging	Very Challenging	Somewhat Challenging	Very Challenging	Somewhat Challenging	Very Challenging	Somewhat Challenging	Very Challenging	Somewhat Challenging	Very Challenging	Somewhat Challenging
Oklahoma		X		X		X		X		X		X		X
Oregon	X		X		X		X		X		X			X
Pennsylvania	X			X		X	X				X		X	
Rhode Island		X		X		X		X		X		X		X
South Carolina		X		X	X		X				X		X	
South Dakota		X	X		X		X		X		X			
Tennessee		X		X		X		X		X		X	X	
Texas		X		X		X	X			X		X	X	
Utah	X			X	X			X		X		X	X	
Vermont	X					X			X			X		X
Virginia		X		X		X		X		X		X	X	
Washington		X				X				X				
West Virginia		X		X		X		X		X		X	X	
Wisconsin		X		X		X		X				X		
Wyoming		X	X		X		X		X		X		X	

Source: OIG analysis of State data collection instrument responses, 2012.

Table A-3. Challenges States Reported With Current Laws and Regulations, by State

	Medicare 1-year timely filing limit		TRICARE 1-year timely filing limit		Lack of enforceable penalties for third parties that refuse to reimburse States		Inability to bill Medicare directly		Lack of rules requiring third parties to reimburse in a timely manner	
State	Very Challenging	Somewhat Challenging	Very Challenging	Somewhat Challenging	Very Challenging	Somewhat Challenging	Very Challenging	Somewhat Challenging	Very Challenging	Somewhat Challenging
Alabama	X		X			X		X		X
Alaska	X			X	X		X			X
Arizona	X		X			X		X		X
Arkansas		X		X	X			X		X
California	X		X		X		X			
Colorado	X		X		X			X		X
Connecticut	X			X		X	X			X
Delaware	X		X			X	X			X
District of Columbia		X		X		X		X		X
Florida	X		X			X	X			X
Georgia		X		X		X	X			X
Hawaii		X		X	X			X		X
Idaho	X		X			X		X		X
Illinois	X			X				X		X
Indiana	X		X			X	X			X
Iowa	X		X			X		X		X
Kansas	X		X			X		X		X
Kentucky	X		X			X		X		X
Louisiana		X	X				X			

Table A-3. (Continued)

	Medicare 1-year timely filing limit		TRICARE 1-year timely filing limit		Lack of enforceable penalties for third parties that refuse to reimburse States		Inability to bill Medicare directly		Lack of rules requiring third parties to reimburse in a timely manner	
State	Very Challenging	Somewhat Challenging	Very Challenging	Somewhat Challenging	Very Challenging	Somewhat Challenging	Very Challenging	Somewhat Challenging	Very Challenging	Somewhat Challenging
Maine	X		X			X		X		X
Maryland		X								
Massachusetts	X		X			X	X			X
Michigan		X		X	X			X	X	
Minnesota		X		X	X					X
Mississippi	X		X		X			X	X	
Missouri	X		X			X		X		X
Montana		X	X			X				
Nebraska		X				X		X		X
Nevada	X		X			X		X		X
New Hampshire	X		X		X		X			
New Jersey	X		X			X		X		X
New Mexico		X		X		X				X
New York	X		X			X		X		X
North Carolina	X		X					X		X
North Dakota		X		X		X		X		X
Ohio		X					X			X
Oklahoma		X		X		X		X		X
Oregon	X		X		X		X			X

State	Medicare 1-year timely filing limit		TRICARE 1-year timely filing limit		Lack of enforceable penalties for third parties that refuse to reimburse States		Inability to bill Medicare directly		Lack of rules requiring third parties to reimburse in a timely manner	
	Very Challenging	Somewhat Challenging	Very Challenging	Somewhat Challenging	Very Challenging	Somewhat Challenging	Very Challenging	Somewhat Challenging	Very Challenging	Somewhat Challenging
Pennsylvania	X		X			X	X			X
Rhode Island		X		X		X		X		X
South Carolina	X		X		X					
South Dakota	X		X		X		X		X	
Tennessee	X		X			X		X		X
Texas	X		X			X	X			
Utah		X		X	X					X
Vermont	X		X				X			
Virginia	X		X			X		X		X
Washington		X			X			X		
West Virginia	X		X			X		X		X
Wisconsin					X		X			X
Wyoming	X		X		X		X		X	

Source: OIG analysis of State data collection instrument responses, 2012.

End Notes

[1] Office of Inspector General (OIG) analysis of U.S. Census Bureau Current Population Survey (CPS) 2008, 2009, and 2010 data (collected in 2009, 2010, and 2011). The CPS is a household survey on employment and unemployment. It also collects data on health insurance coverage.

[2] Ibid.

[3] OIG, Medicaid Recovery of Pharmacy Payments From Liable Third Parties, OEI-03-00-00030, August 2001.

[4] GAO, Medicaid Third-Party Liability: Federal Guidance Needed to Help States Address Continuing Problems, GAO-06-862, September 2006.

[5] Centers for Medicare & Medicaid Services (CMS), State Medicaid Manual, Pub. No. 45, ch. 3, § 3900.1.

[6] In a few limited circumstances, Medicaid is not the payer of last resort. For example, Ryan White programs are the payer of last resort, even with respect to Medicaid. Ryan White Comprehensive AIDS Resources Emergency Act of 1990, P.L. 101-381, § 2615; 42 U.S.C. 300ff-25.

[7] Social Security Act § 1902(a)(25), 42 U.S.C. § 1396a(a)(25).

[8] CMS, State Medicaid Director Letter, December 15, 2006 (SMD #06-026), Questions and Answers. Accessed at http://downloads.cms.gov/cmsgov/archiveddownloads/SMDL/downloads/SMD121506QandA.pdf on August 29, 2012.

[9] CMS, State Medicaid Manual, Pub. No. 45, ch. 3, § 3901.

[10] Social Security Act § 1902(a)(25), 42 U.S.C. § 1396a(a)(25).

[11] 42 CFR § 433.138; CMS, State Medicaid Manual, Pub. No. 45, §§ 3902 and 3903.

[12] 42 CFR § 433.139(b).

[13] Because Medicaid beneficiaries assign to the States any rights they may have to support or payment from a liable third party, States are able to pay and chase claims if a third party awards retroactive coverage. Instances in which Medicaid beneficiaries may obtain retroactive health coverage from a liable third party include court-ordered health coverage and Medicare retroactive eligibility.

[14] Social Security Act §§ 1902(a)(25)(E) and (F), 42 U.S.C. §§ 1396a(a)(25)(E) and (F). See also 42 CFR § 433.139(b)(3).

[15] Office of Management and Budget, Fiscal Year 2013 Budget of the U.S. Government: Cuts, Consolidations, and Savings. Accessed at http://www.whitehouse.gov/sites/default/files/omb/budget/fy2013/assets/ccs.pdf on August 29, 2012.

[16] Arkansas Dept. of Health and Human Services v. Ahlborn, 547 U.S. 268 (2006).

[17] 42 CFR § 433.151. Pursuant to 42 CFR § 433.151, States must enter into written cooperative agreements for enforcement of rights to and collection of third-party benefits with at least one of the following entities: State child support enforcement agency, any appropriate agency of any State, and appropriate courts and law enforcement officials. Collections through cooperative agreements are a specific line item on the CMS-64.9A.

[18] 42 CFR § 433.13 (f)(2).

[19] Ibid.

[20] 42 CFR § 430.30(c); CMS, State Medicaid Manual, Pub. No. 45, § 2500(A)(1).

[21] DRA, P.L. 109-171 § 6035(a), amending Social Security Act § 1902(a)(25), 42 U.S.C. § 1396a(a)(25).

[22] DRA, P.L. 109-171 § 6035(b)(3), amending Social Security Act § 1902(a)(25), 42 U.S.C. § 1396a(a)(25). See also CMS, State Medicaid Director Letter, December 15, 2006 (SMD

#06-026), Questions and Answers. Accessed at http://downloads.cms.gov/cmsgov/archived-downloads/SMDL/downloads/SMD121506QandA.pdf on August 29, 2012.

[23] DRA, P.L. 109-171, § 6035(c), 42 U.S.C. § 1396a note.

[24] ACA, P.L. 111-148 § 6404, amending Social Security Act §§ 1814(a)(1), 1835(a)(1), and 1842(b)(3)(B), 42 U.S.C. §§ 1395f(a)(1), 1395u(b)(3)(B), and 1395n(a). The Secretary may specify exceptions to the 1 calendar year period under each provision.

[25] If the Medicare contractor determines that CMS's conditions for the exception are met, it may allow the provider a filing extension from the end of the sixth calendar month from the month in which States recovered their money. See CMS, Medicare Claims Processing Manual, Pub. No. 100-04, ch.1, § 70.7.3.

[26] 32 CFR § 199.7(d). TRICARE was formerly known as the Civilian Health and Medical Program of the Uniformed Services and is still referred to as such in some regulations.

[27] OIG, Medicaid Recovery of Pharmacy Payments From Liable Third Parties.

[28] Ibid.

[29] GAO, Medicaid Third-Party Liability: Federal Guidance Needed to Help States Address Continuing Problems. The data in the report were collected prior to the DRA's effective date, although the report was published after the effective date.

[30] Ibid.

[31] All data collected directly from States also reflect both the Federal and State share.

[32] To account for inflation, we used the Consumer Price Index conversion factor to convert to 2011 dollars.

[33] To calculate a reasonable estimate of the amount that States might be able to recover from casualty insurance and probated estates, we adjusted the raw numbers provided by States by the rates of return for closed cases (data also provided by States).

[34] The remaining seven States did not provide this information.

[35] OIG analysis of U.S. Census Bureau CPS 2008, 2009, and 2010 data (collected in 2009, 2010, and 2011).

[36] Each State determined what dollars were at risk of not being recovered using its own methodology. As a result, this amount represents varying time periods.

[37] DRA, P.L. 109-171 § 6035, Social Security Act § 1902(a)(25), 42 U.S.C. § 1396a.

[38] OIG, Medicaid Recovery of Pharmacy Payments From Liable Third Parties.

[39] GAO, Medicaid Third-Party Liability: Federal Guidance Needed to Help States Address Continuing Problems.

[40] OIG, Medicaid Recovery of Pharmacy Payments From Liable Third Parties.

[41] GAO, Medicaid Third-Party Liability: Federal Guidance Needed to Help States Address Continuing Problems.

[42] See Table A-1 in Appendix A for a list of these challenges by State.

[43] 45 CFR § 164.506.

[44] CMS, State Medicaid Director Letter, June 21, 2010 (SMDL #10-011), Questions and Answers. Accessed at http://downloads.cms.gov/cmsgov/archiveddownloads/SMDL/downloads/SMD10011.pdf on August 29, 2012.

[45] OIG, Medicaid Recovery of Pharmacy Payments From Liable Third Parties.

[46] CMS, State Medicaid Director Letter, December 15, 2006 (SMD #06-026), Questions and Answers. Accessed at http://downloads.cms.gov/cmsgov/archiveddownloads/SMDL/downloads/SMD121506QandA.pdf on August 29, 2012.

[47] OIG, Medicaid Recovery of Pharmacy Payments From Liable Third Parties.

[48] GAO, Medicaid Third-Party Liability: Federal Guidance Needed to Help States Address Continuing Problems.

[49] See Table A-2 in Appendix A for a list of these challenges by State.
[50] See, e.g., Caremark, Inc. v. Goetz, 480 F.3d 779 (6th Cir. 2007).
[51] Ibid.
[52] Ibid.
[53] See Table A-3 in Appendix A for a list of these challenges by State.
[54] 42 CFR 424.44(b)(2).
[55] CMS, Modifying Timely Filing Exceptions on Retroactive Medicare Entitlement and Retroactive Medicare Entitlement Involving State Medicaid Agencies, Medicare Claims Processing Manual (CMS Pub. 100-04), Transmittal 2477, Change Request 7834 (May 25, 2012; effective August 27, 2012). Accessed at http://www.cms.gov/Regulations-and-Guidance/Guidance/Transmittals/downloads/R2477CP.pdf on August 29, 2012.
[56] 32 CFR § 199.7(d).
[57] TRICARE, TRICARE Reimbursement Manual 6010.58-M, ch. 1, § 20, para. 2.1.2 (Feb. 1, 2008).
[58] TRICARE, TRICARE Reimbursement Manual 6010.58-M, ch. 1, add. A (Feb. 1, 2008).

In: Medicaid Third-Party Liability
Editor: Donald Murphy

ISBN: 978-1-63483-049-2

Chapter 3

COORDINATION OF BENEFITS AND THIRD-PARTY LIABILITY (COB/TPL) IN THE MEDICAID PROGRAM: A GUIDE TO EFFECTIVE STATE AGENCY PRACTICES*

Centers for Medicare & Medicaid Services

INTRODUCTION

The intent of this Effective Practices Guide is to provide state Medicaid agencies with information on practices that could assist states in improving their identification and successful pursuit of legally liable third party resources. Each practice included in the guide has proven to be effective for the submitting state. State agencies that consider adopting any of these practices should assess whether the practice is transferable to their own state operations. A contact person is listed for each practice and will be available to discuss the practice in greater detail with a state that considers adopting the practice.

The Effective Practices Guide was developed in response to a recommendation by the Office of the Inspector General ((OIG), U.S. Department of Health and Human Services, following on a study of Medicaid COB/TPL

* This is an edited, reformatted and augmented version of a report issued by the Department of Health and Human Services, July 2014.

savings from 2001 to 2011 ("Medicaid Third-Party Liability Savings Increased, but Challenges Remain", OEI-05-11-00130, issued January 2013). The study determined trends in Medicaid TPL savings during that period and gathered information from states regarding challenges and issues the states faced in trying to identify third party coverage and recover payments from liable third parties.

The Guide provides an opportunity for peer assistance among the state Medicaid programs through sharing of practices that are in place, and working, in the states in December 2013. The Guide includes effective practices to address some of the challenges and issues identified in the OIG study, and other challenges to maximizing third party savings.

EFFECTIVE STATE PRACTICES, BY TOPIC AND SUBMITTING STATES

1. States' Interactions with Health Insurers: Iowa, Michigan, Mississippi, New York, Ohio, Texas, Washington
2. Health Insurance Portability and Accountability Act (HIPAA): Iowa
3. States' Interactions with Pharmacy Benefits Managers (PBMs): Iowa, Minnesota
4. Other Third Party Liability Topics: Oklahoma, Pennsylvania, Washington

Effective practices follow, listed by state.

IOWA

Issue:	Denials from third parties for procedural reasons Denials from third parties with no explanation Third parties not responding when State submits bills Third parties not abiding by 3-year timely filing rules Third-party documentation submitted with reimbursement does not indicate which claims are being reimbursed Third parties not accepting States' right to collect Pharmacy benefit managers claim they do not have the authority to reimburse States directly Third party concerns about the Health Insurance Portability and Accountability Act of 1996 and releasing insurance coverage information to states

<table>
<tr><td colspan="2">Confusing or incomplete Explanation of Benefits forms from third parties
Cooperation from pharmacy benefit managers</td></tr>
<tr><td>IN THE RESPONDING STATE, THIS ISSUE:

__X__CURRENTLY OCCURS OR HAS OCCURRED:
____VERY FREQUENTLY
__X__OFTEN ENOUGH TO REQUIRE CORRECTION
____INFREQUENTLY
____DOESN'T OCCUR OR HASN'T OCCURRED</td><td>EFFECT OF THE PRACTICE:

__X__RESOLVED THE ISSUE FULLY
____ RESOLVED THE ISSUE PARTIALLY (Indicate what was resolved and what remains in the Summary below.)
____RESOLVED TEMPORARILY WITH A WORKAROUND PROCESS</td></tr>
<tr><td colspan="2">WHY DOES THIS ISSUE OCCUR?
Insurance carriers do not follow the Deficit Reduction Act or Iowa legislation 249A.37.</td></tr>
<tr><td colspan="2">SUMMARY OF EFFECTIVE PRACTICE:

Some insurance carriers did not effectively adopt and implement the provisions of the Deficit Reduction Act (DRA) of 2005 - indicating that Iowa did not have specific state legislation to support the DRA. In response, Iowa passed specific legislation to support the DRA as it pertains to doing business in Iowa. This legislation is codified in the Code of Iowa at 249A.37. The legislation addresses the following;
Service benefit plans, managed care organizations, pharmacy benefits managers, and other parties that are, by statute, contract, or agreement, legally responsible for payment of a claim for a health care item or service.
The statutory language states:

249A.37 HEALTH CARE INFORMATION SHARING.

1. As a condition of doing business in the state, health insurers including self-insured plans, group health plans as defined in the federal Employee Retirement Income Security Act of 1974, Pub. L. No. 93-406, service benefit plans, managed care organizations, pharmacy benefits managers, and other parties that are, by statute, contract, or agreement, legally responsible for payment of a claim for a health care item or service, shall do all of the following:</td></tr>
</table>

a. Provide, with respect to individuals who are eligible for or are provided medical assistance under the state's medical assistance state plan, upon the request of the state, information to determine during what period the individual or the individual's spouse or dependents may be or may have been covered by a health insurer and the nature of the coverage that is or was provided by the health insurer, including the name, address, and identifying number of the plan, in accordance with section 505.25, in a manner prescribed by the department of human services or as agreed upon by the department and the entity specified in this section. b. Accept the state's right of recovery and the assignment to the state of any right of an individual or other entity to payment from the party for an item or service for which payment has been made under the medical assistance state plan. c. Respond to any inquiry by the state regarding a claim for payment for any health care item or service that is submitted no later than three years after the date of the provision of such health care item or service. d. Agree not to deny any claim submitted by the state solely on the basis of the date of submission of the claim, the type or format of the claim form, or a failure to present proper documentation at the point-of-sale that is the basis of the claim, if all of the following conditions are met: (1) The claim is submitted to the entity by the state within the three-year period beginning on the date on which the item or service was furnished. (2) Any action by the state to enforce its rights with respect to such claim is commenced within six years of the date that the claim was submitted by the state. 2. The department of human services may adopt rules pursuant to chapter 17A as necessary to implement this section. Rules governing the exchange of information under this section shall be consistent with all laws, regulations, and rules relating to the confidentiality or privacy of personal information or medical records, including but not limited to the federal Health Insurance Portability and Accountability Act of 1996, Pub. L. No. 104-191, and regulations promulgated in accordance with that Act and published in 45 C.F.R.
SPECIAL FACTORS THAT SUPPORT THE EFFECTIVE PRACTICE: (Ex: State Law, Case Law, Data Exchange Agreements, Data Systems, Contractor Use, etc.) The State of Iowa contracts pay and chase activities to an external vendor. This includes post pay and chase billing follow-up; we call this Local Yield Management.

Iowa has dedicated staff devoted primarily to challenging carriers for what appear to be inappropriate denials and to respond to requests for additional information. We find that one-on-one education and follow-up helps the carrier process claims correctly. More examples of yield management activitiesinclude: 1) Follow-up with carriers to get a clear understanding of certain claim denials on the Explanation of Benefits (EOB's). 2) Review with carriers the practice of denying claims for procedural reasons. 3) Carriers are contacted when no response is received on a reclamation claim. 4) If a carrier denies a reclamation claim due to needing additional information from a provider, our Local Yield Management team get the information needed in order for the claim to process. In State Fiscal Year 2013 Local Yield Management staff was able to recover $8,905,715.00 Iowa will be tracking the yield management separately from pay and chase recovery work on a going basis to monitor progress in the reduction of improper Medicaid claim denials.
FOR MORE INFORMATION, CONTACT: (Name and Title, Phone Number, Email Address) Sara Schneider Iowa Department of Human Services Iowa Medicaid Enterprise(IME)/Bureau of Adult and Children's Medical Programs Phone: 515-974-3281 E-mail: sschnei@dhs.state.ia.us

MICHIGAN

ISSUE: Lack of enforceable penalties for third parties that refuse to reimburse States	
IN THE RESPONDING STATE, THIS ISSUE: ____CURRENTLY OCCURS OR HAS OCCURRED: ____VERY FREQUENTLY ____OFTEN ENOUGH TO	EFFECT OF PROMISING PRACTICE: __ X _RESOLVED THE ISSUE FULLY ____RESOLVED THE ISSUE PARTIALLY (Indicate what

REQUIRE CORRECTION ____INFREQUENTLY __ X __DOESN'T OCCUR OR HASN'T OCCURED	was resolved and what remains in the Summary below.) ____RESOLVED TEMPORARILY WITH A WORKAROUND PROCESS
WHY DOES THIS ISSUE OCCUR? Medical third party declines or delays rightful reimbursement for services that were paid by Medicaid but were services in which the medical third party was responsible as the primary payer.	
SUMMARY OF PROMISING PRACTICE: Section 7 of Act 593 allows for a punitive penalty of $500 for every day the medical third party refuses to fulfill a recovery request from Third Party Liability. The Act gives the medical third party the right to appeal the penalty through the administrative law process in the State. The Third Party Liability Division has the full support from the Office of Legal Affairs, giving the Act the legal support necessary for enforcement. SHARING HEALTH CARE INFORMATION ACT Act 593 of 2006 AN ACT to provide for the sharing of certain health care coverage information; to provide for the powers and duties of certain departments and agencies; and to provide penalties and fines. History: 2006, Act 593, Imd. Eff. Jan. 3, 2007 The People of the State of Michigan enact: 550.281 Definitions. Sec. 1. As used in this act: (a) "Department" means the department of community health. (b) "Entity" means a health insurer; a health maintenance organization; a nonprofit health care corporation; a managed care corporation; a preferred provider organization; an organization operating pursuant to the prudent purchaser act, 1984 PA 233, MCL 550.51 to 550.63; a self-funded health plan; a professional association, trust, pool, union, or fraternal group, offering health coverage; a system of health care delivery and financing operating pursuant to section 3573 of the insurance code of 1956, 1956 PA 218, MCL 500.3573; and a third party administrator. (c) "Medical assistance" means the medical assistance program administered by the state under the social welfare act, 1939 PA 280, MCL 400.1 to 400.119b.	

(d) "Qualified health plan" means that term as defined in section 111i of the social welfare act, 1939 PA 280, MCL 400.111i.
History: 2006, Act 593, Imd. Eff. Jan. 3, 2007
550.283 Determination that health coverage recipient is also medical assistance recipient; information to be provided by health insurer.
Sec. 3.
(1) An entity shall provide on a monthly basis to the department, in a format determined by the department, information necessary to enable the department or entity to determine whether a health coverage recipient of the entity is also a medical assistance recipient.
(2) If a health coverage recipient of the entity is also a medical assistance recipient, the entity shall do all of the following by not later than 180 days after the department's request:
(a) Pay the department for, or assign to the department any right of recovery owed to the entity for, a covered health claim for which medical assistance payment has been made.
(b) Respond to any inquiry by the department concerning a claim for payment for any health care item or service that is submitted not later than 3 years after the date the health care item or service was provided.
(3) An entity shall not deny a claim submitted by the department solely on the basis of the date of submission of the claim, the type or format of the claim form, or a failure to present proper documentation at the time the health care item or service that is the basis of the claim was provided so long as both of the following apply:
(a) The claim is submitted to the entity within 3 years of the date that the health care item or service that is the subject of the claim was provided.
(b) Any action by the state to enforce its rights under this subdivision is commenced within 6 years of the date that the health care item or service that is the subject of the claim was provided.
History: 2006, Act 593, Imd. Eff. Jan. 3, 2007
550.285 Determination that health coverage recipient is also medical assistance recipient; actions by department.
Sec. 5.
If the department determines that a health coverage recipient is also a medical assistance recipient:
(a) The department may use information received under section 3 to update the medical assistance database maintained by the department.
(b) If the medical assistance recipient is covered by a qualified health plan, the department shall share with that qualified health plan all information received under this act by the department for that medical assistance recipient.
History: 2006, Act 593, Imd. Eff. Jan. 3, 2007

550.287 Violation of act; administrative fine; notice; right to hearing. Sec. 7. *An entity that violates this act is subject to an administrative fine of not more than $500.00 for each day the entity does not comply with section 3(1) or with a request for information made pursuant to section 3(2).* Upon the department's determination that a violation of this act has occurred, the entity has a right to notice of the alleged violation and an opportunity for a hearing under the administrative procedures act of 1969, 1969 PA 306, MCL 24.201 to 24.328. History: 2006, Act 593, Imd. Eff. Jan. 3, 2007 550.289 Rules. Sec. 9. The department may promulgate rules pursuant to the administrative procedures act of 1969, 1969 PA 306, MCL 24.201 to 24.328, necessary to implement this act. Rules governing the exchange of information under this act shall be consistent with all laws, regulations, and rules relating to the confidentiality or privacy of personal information or medical records, including, but not limited to, the health insurance portability and accountability act of 1996, Public Law 104-191, and regulations promulgated under that act, 45 CFR parts 160 to 164. History: 2006, Act 593, Imd. Eff. Jan. 3, 2007
SPECIAL FACTORS THAT SUPPORT THE PROMISING PRACTICE: (Ex: State Law, Case Law, Data Exchange Agreements, Data Systems, Contractor Use, etc.) State Law
FOR MORE INFORMATION, CONTACT: (Name and Title, Phone Number, Email Address) Tanya Lowers Director of Third Party Liability 517-335-8989 lowerst@michigan.gov

MINNESOTA

ISSUE: Pharmacy Benefit Managers claim they do not have the authority to reimburse states directly.	
IN THE RESPONDING STATE, THIS ISSUE: ____CURRENTLY OCCURS OR HAS OCCURRED: _ X ___VERY FREQUENTLY ____OFTEN ENOUGH TO REQUIRE	*EFFECT OF THE PRACTICE:* ____RESOLVED THE ISSUE FULLY ____RESOLVED THE ISSUE PARTIALLY (*Indicate what was resolved and what remains in the Summary below.*)

CORRECTION ____INFREQUENTLY ____DOESN'T OCCUR OR HASN'T OCCURRED	_ X ___RESOLVED TEMPORARILY WITH A WORKAROUND PROCESS
WHY DOES THIS ISSUE OCCUR? The employer/insurance company has not given Permission to the PBM to pay claims directly to Medicaid.	
SUMMARY OF EFFECTIVE PRACTICE: We send a letter to the employer or insurance company asking them to contact the PBM and give them whatever authority they need in order to process the claims. The letter advises the employer/insurance company that they are ultimately responsible for payment of the covered services.	
SPECIAL FACTORS THAT SUPPORT THE EFFECTIVE PRACTICE: (Ex: State Law, Case Law, Data Exchange Agreements, Data Systems, Contractor Use, etc.)	
FOR MORE INFORMATION, CONTACT: (Name and Title, Phone Number, Email Address) Pat Dault-Beauchane Supervisor, Health Insurance Recovery Unit Benefit Recovery Section 651-431-3138 651-431-7431 (Fax) Pat.dault-beauchane@state.mn.us Sandy Burge Manager, Benefit Recovery Section 651-431-3284 651-431-7431 (Fax) Sandy.burge@state.mn.us	

MINNESOTA

ISSUE: Pharmacy providers who submit erroneous denial/reject reason	
IN THE RESPONDING STATE, THIS ISSUE: ____CURRENTLY OCCURS OR HAS OCCURRED: _ X ___VERY FREQUENTLY ____OFTEN ENOUGH TO REQUIRE CORRECTION	*EFFECT OF THE PRACTICE:* ____RESOLVED THE ISSUE FULLY ____RESOLVED THE ISSUE PARTIALLY (*Indicate what was resolved and what remains in the Summary below.*)

____INFREQUENTLY ____DOESN'T OCCUR OR HASN'T OCCURRED	_ X ___RESOLVED TEMPORARILY WITH A WORKAROUND PROCESS

WHY DOES THIS ISSUE OCCUR?

Pharmacies submit claims with erroneous TPL information. In some instances the PBMs deny the claims for 1) no prior authorization, 2) brand name drug dispensed and should have used a generic ,3) drug should have been dispensed by a specialty pharmacy. In these cases, the pharmacy submits a claim with a reason code stating the drug is not covered. In Minnesota, we pay and chase all pharmacy claims for clients who have reported insurance, but do not show a payment from the TPL. It has been our experience that the PBMs deny our claims 1) without an explanation, 2) as duplicates, or 3) they don't respond at all.

SUMMARY OF EFFECTIVE PRACTICE:

We recently started auditing the claims before we submit them to the carriers. We review claims with larger dollar amounts and call the PBM for additional information. This seems to work better than sending them a claim. If the PBM gives us information that: 1) a prior authorization is needed, 2) a generic should have been dispensed, or 3) a specialty Pharmacy should have been used, we take the money back from the provider as being erroneously billed.
The first week we did this, we took back in excess of $60,000.00.

SPECIAL FACTORS THAT SUPPORT THE EFFECTIVE PRACTICE:

(Ex: State Law, Case Law, Data Exchange Agreements, Data Systems, Contractor Use, etc.)

FOR MORE INFORMATION, CONTACT:

(Name and Title, Phone Number, Email Address)
Pat Dault-Beauchane,
Supervisor, Health Insurance Recovery Unit Benefit Recovery Section 651-431-3138
651-431-7431 (Fax)
Pat.dault-beauchane@state.mn.us
Or
Sandy Burge
Manager, Benefit Recovery Section 651-431-3284 651-431-7431 (Fax)
Sandy.burge@state.mn.us

MISSISSIPPI

ISSUE: Accept Medicaid 's right of recovery and not deny claims submitted by the Division	
IN THE RESPONDING STATE, THIS ISSUE: _X___CURRENTLY OCCURS OR HAS OCCURRED: ____VERY FREQUENTLY ____OFTEN ENOUGH TO REQUIRE CORRECTION ____INFREQUENTLY ____DOESN'T OCCUR OR HASN'T OCCURRED	EFFECT OF PRACTICE: _X __RESOLVED THE ISSUE FULLY ____RESOLVED THE ISSUE PARTIALLY (Indicate what was resolved and what remains in the Summary below.) ____RESOLVED TEMPORARILY WITH A WORKAROUND PROCESS
WHY DOES THIS ISSUE OCCUR? Third party denies claims submitted by Medicaid on the basis of certain errors as condition of doing business in Mississippi.	
SUMMARY OF EFFECTIVE PRACTICE: § 43-13-126. Health insurers required to provide certain information to the Division of Medicaid, accept Division's right of recovery and not deny claims submitted by Division on the basis of certain errors as condition of doing business in Mississippi. As a condition of doing business in the state, health insurers, including self-insured plans, group health plans (as defined in Section 607(1) of the Employee Retirement Income Security Act of 1974), service benefit plans, managed care organizations, pharmacy benefit managers, or other parties that are by statute, contract, or agreement, legally responsible for payment of a claim for a health care item or service, are required to: (a) Provide, with respect to individuals who are eligible for, or are provided, medical assistance under the state plan, upon the request of the Division of Medicaid, information to determine during what period the individual or their dependents may be (or may have been) covered by the health insurer and the nature of the coverage that is or was provided by the health insurer (including the name, address and identifying number of the plan) in a manner prescribed by the Secretary of the Department of Health and Human Services; (b) Accept the Division of Medicaid's right of recovery and the assignment to the division of any right of an individual or other entity to payment from the party for an item or service for which payment has been made under the	

state plan; (c) Respond to any inquiry by the Division of Medicaid regarding a claim for payment for any health care item or service that is submitted not later than three (3) years after the date of the provision of that health care item or service; and (d) Agree not to deny a claim submitted by the Division of Medicaid solely on the basis of the date of submission of the claim, the type or format of the claim form, or a failure to present proper documentation at the point-of-sale that is the claim, if: (i) The claim is submitted by the division within the three-year period beginning on the date on which the item or service was furnished; and (ii) Any action by the division to enforce its rights with respect to the claim is begun within six (6) years of the division's submission of the claim.
SPECIAL FACTORS THAT SUPPORT THE EFFECTIVE PRACTICE: (Ex: State Law, Case Law, Data Exchange Agreements, Data Systems, Contractor Use, etc.) Laws, 2007, ch. 553, § 3, eff. from and after July1, 2007. FOR MORE INFORMATION, CONTACT: (Name and Title, Phone Number, Email Address) Margaret Robinson, Office Director II, 601-359-6113, Margaret.robinson@medicaid.ms.gov

NEW YORK

ISSUE: Denials for Prior Authorization	
IN THE RESPONDING STATE, THIS ISSUE: __ X __CURRENTLY OCCURS OR HAS OCCURRED: ____VERY FREQUENTLY __ X __OFTEN ENOUGH TO REQUIRE CORRECTION ____INFREQUENTLY ____DOESN'T OCCUR OR HASN'T OCCURRED	*EFFECT OF THE PRACTICE:* ____RESOLVED THE ISSUE FULLY __ X __RESOLVED THE ISSUE PARTIALLY (*Indicate what was resolved and what remains in the Summary below.*) ____RESOLVED TEMPORARILY WITH A WORKAROUND PROCESS
WHY DOES THIS ISSUE OCCUR? Commercial Insurance carriers deny Medicaid Subrogation claims for not having prior authorization to receive treatment.	
SUMMARY OF EFFECTIVE PRACTICE:	

Referring to The Federal law (42 U.S.C. 1396a(a)(25)(A)), subsequent NY State Insurance and Social Services Law, and in partnership with our TPL vendor, the NY Office of the Medicaid Inspector General (OMIG) appeals all denials for prior authorization. The body of the letter sent with the appeal includes the following: In accordance with §3212(e)(3) (C) of New York State Insurance Law, such a denial is not permitted for Medicaid subrogation claims. §3212(e)(3) (C) reads as follows: *"An insurer shall not deny a claim made in conformance with paragraph (b) of subdivision two of section three hundred sixty-seven-a of the social services law solely on the basis of the date of submission of the claim, the type or format of the claim form, or a failure to present proper documentation at the point-of-sale that is the basis of the claim."* §367-A(2) of the New York State Social Services Law, referenced above section of the NYS Insurance Law, reads as follows: *"Liable third parties shall not deny a claim made by a social services official or the department in conformance with this paragraph solely on the basis of the date of submission of the claim, the type or format of the claim form, or a failure to present proper documentation at the point-of-sale that is the basis of the claim."* Please re-process these claims and respond promptly with either payment or a valid denial.
SPECIAL FACTORS THAT SUPPORT THE EFFECTIVE PRACTICE:
FOR MORE INFORMATION, CONTACT: (Name and Title, Phone Number, Email Address) Larry Matthews, 518-474-8347, Lawrence.Matthews@omig.ny.gov

OHIO

ISSUE: Denials from third parties for procedural reasons	
IN THE RESPONDING STATE, THIS ISSUE: __X__CURRENTLY OCCURS OR HAS OCCURRED: ____VERY FREQUENTLY ____OFTEN ENOUGH TO REQUIRE CORRECTION __X__INFREQUENTLY ____DOESN'T OCCUR OR HASN'T	*EFFECT OF PROMISING PRACTICE:* _X___RESOLVED THE ISSUE FULLY ____RESOLVED THE ISSUE PARTIALLY (*Indicate what was resolved and what remains in the Summary below.*) ____RESOLVED TEMPORARILY

OCCURRED	WITH A WORKAROUND PROCESS

WHY DOES THIS ISSUE OCCUR?
Some insurance carriers are not familiar with the Deficit Reduction Act of 2005 or Ohio legislation.

SUMMARY OF PROMISING PRACTICE:

Even after the implementation of the Deficit Reduction Act language in Ohio law, some insurance carriers would deny Medicaid reclamation claims for not obtaining prior authorization. To address this issue, Ohio passed specific legislation in 2009 to specifically outline a claim could not be denied for lack of obtaining prior authorization. This legislation applies to fee for service as well as Medicare Managed Care organizations. Ohio also increased the timeframe to six years for its right of recovery. The legislation in Ohio is-

5101.573 Third-party duties - managed care organizations.

(A) Subject to divisions (B) and (C) of this section, a third party shall do all of the following:

(1) Accept the department of job and family services' right of recovery under section 5101.58 of the Revised Code and the assignment of rights to the department that are described in section 5101.59 of the Revised Code;

(2) Respond to an inquiry by the department regarding a claim for payment of a medical item or service that was submitted to the third party not later than six years after the date of the provision of such medical item or service;

(3) Not charge a fee to do either of the following for a claim described in division (A)(2) of this section:

a) Determine whether the claim should be paid;

b) Process the claim.

(4) Pay a claim described in division (A)(2) of this section;

(5) Not deny a claim submitted by the department solely on the basis of the date of submission of the claim, type or format of the claim form, or a failure by the medical assistance recipient who is the subject of the claim to present proper documentation of coverage at the time of service, if both of the following are true:

The claim was submitted by the department not later than six years after the date of the provision of the medical item or service.

An action by the department to enforce its right of recovery under section 5101.58 of the Revised Code on the claim was commenced not later than six years after the department's submission of the claim.

Consider the department's payment of a claim for a medical item or service to be the equivalent of the medical assistance recipient having obtained prior authorization for the item or service from the third party;

Not deny a claim described in division (A)(6) of this section that is submitted by the department solely on the basis of the medical assistance recipient's failure to obtain prior authorization for the medical item or service.

(B) For purposes of the requirements in division (A) of this section, a third party shall treat a managed care organization as the department for a claim in which both of the following are true:

The individual who is the subject of the claim received a medical item or service through a managed care organization that has entered into a contract with the department of job and family services under section 5111.17 of the Revised Code;

The department has assigned its right of recovery for the claim to the managed care organization.

(C) The time limitations associated with the requirements in divisions (A)(2) and (5) of this section apply only to submissions of claims to,
and payments of claims by, a health insurer to which 42 U.S.C. 1396a(a)(25)(I) applies.

Amended by 129th General Assembly File No. 28, HB 153, § 101.01, eff. 9/29/2011.

Amended by 128th General Assembly File No. 9, HB 1, § 101.01, eff. 10/16/2009.

Effective Date: 2007 HB119 09-29-2007

Lawriter - ORC - 5101.573 Third-party duties - managed care organizations.

Page 1 of 1

http://

SPECIAL FACTORS THAT SUPPORT THE PROMISING PRACTICE:

(Ex: State Law, Case Law, Data Exchange Agreements, Data Systems, Contractor Use, etc.)

Ohio's TPL pay and chase vendor tracked by year the impact of the denials based on reason that claims were denied for lack of prior authorization. Note the large reduction in the denial reason in SFY 2012.

OH Denial Analysis - No Prior Authorization: Denials

Based	on date of	service
SFY	Total No. of Claims	Total Medicaid Paid Amounts
2000	39	$1,249.81
2001	81	$21,704.96
2002	1,880	$253,110.78
2003	7,034	$1,236,309.71
2004	9,708	$1,329,234.24

2005	10,237	$1,751,869.57
2006	7,224	$1,321,521.05
2007	8,940	$1,330,381.91
2008	9,717	$1,308,828.46
2009	9,913	$1,612,121.00
2010	6,402	$1,113,844.68
2011	7,910	$1,252,648.27
2012	2,526	$889,697.02
2013	1,086	$503,857.17
Total	82,697	$13,926,378.63

FOR MORE INFORMATION, CONTACT: (Name and Title, Phone Number, Email Address) Patrick A. Tighe Patrick.Tighe@medicaid.ohio.gov 614-752-3635

OKLAHOMA

ISSUE: Not passing legislation that is not mandated, but will enhance the Medicaid program	
IN THE RESPONDING STATE, THIS ISSUE: _ X ___CURRENTLY OCCURS OR HAS OCCURRED: ____VERY FREQUENTLY ____OFTEN ENOUGH TO REQUIRE CORRECTION ____INFREQUENTLY ____DOESN'T OCCUR OR HASN'T OCCURRED	*EFFECT OF PRACTICE:* ____RESOLVED THE ISSUE FULLY ____RESOLVED THE ISSUE PARTIALLY (*Indicate what was resolved and what remains in the Summary below.*) __ X __RESOLVED TEMPORARILY WITH A WORKAROUND PROCESS
WHY DOES THIS ISSUE OCCUR? When legislation is not mandated, it is sometimes not seen as a priority or important.	
SUMMARY OF EFFECTIVE PRACTICE: This may not happen as regularly anymore, but we have found that in our state it is fairly easy to pass legislation when things are required to be in compliance with Federal law, i.e. DRA, ACA etc. We have learned that during this time, we should take advantage of the situation and put in any language that we have been	

trying to pass to ride on the coattails of the "required changes". Doing this has resulted in the passing of many laws that enhanced the Medicaid program.
SPECIAL FACTORS THAT SUPPORT THE EFFECTIVE PRACTICE: (Ex: State Law, Case Law, Data Exchange Agreements, Data Systems, Contractor Use, etc.) Federal Law
FOR MORE INFORMATION, CONTACT: (Name and Title, Phone Number, Email Address) Susan Geyer Business Process Manager (405)522-7199 Susan.geyer@okhca.org

OKLAHOMA

ISSUE: Medicaid applicants' health insurance coverage was not being captured on the online eligibility application.	
IN THE RESPONDING STATE, THIS ISSUE: __ X __CURRENTLY OCCURS OR HAS OCCURRED: ____VERY FREQUENTLY ____OFTEN ENOUGH TO REQUIRE CORRECTION ____INFREQUENTLY ____DOESN'T OCCUR OR HASN'T OCCURRED	*EFFECT OF PRACTICE:* _ X ___RESOLVED THE ISSUE FULLY ____RESOLVED THE ISSUE PARTIALLY (*Indicate what was resolved and what remains in the Summary below.*) ____RESOLVED TEMPORARILY WITH A WORKAROUND PROCESS
WHY DOES THIS ISSUE OCCUR? Because TPL was not brought to the table early in the process of establishing an on-line enrollment application.	
SUMMARY OF EFFECTIVE PRACTICE: Work with the system as you begin the process of establishing on-line enrollment to insure that TPL has a place at the table. It is imperative that you make system designers aware of TPL's needs from the beginning of the process. After it is built, it is too late. Also, I would highly recommend drop-down menus for things like carrier name, and not allowing free- form text as much as possible. That will allow for automated update if you choose that option in the future.	

SPECIAL FACTORS THAT SUPPORT THE EFFECTIVE PRACTICE: (Ex: State Law, Case Law, Data Exchange Agreements, Data Systems, Contractor Use, etc.)
FOR MORE INFORMATION, CONTACT: (Name and Title, Phone Number, Email Address) Susan Geyer Business Process Manager (405)522-7199 Susan.geyer@okhca.org

PENNSYLVANIA

ISSUE: Coordination of benefits of deemed newborns, when either parent has other insurance coverage. Providing for health and welfare of newborn children and their parents by regulating certain health insurance coverage for newborn children.	
IN THE RESPONDING STATE, THIS ISSUE: __X__CURRENTLY OCCURS OR HAS OCCURRED: _X_VERY FREQUENTLY ____OFTEN ENOUGH TO REQUIRE CORRECTION ____INFREQUENTLY DOESN'T OCCUR OR HASN'T OCCURRED	*EFFECT OF PRACTICE:* ____RESOLVED THE ISSUE FULLY __X__RESOLVED THE ISSUE PARTIALLY (Indicate what was resolved and what remains in the Summary below.) ____RESOLVED TEMPORARILY WITH A WORKAROUND PROCESS
WHY DOES THIS ISSUE OCCUR? Interpretation, by insurance carriers, of federal and Pennsylvania state laws for insurance carrier liability with continued confinement of the newborn past the mandated period of 48/96 hours. The Newborns' and Mothers' Health Protection Act states that carriers pay for at least 48-hours (for vaginal delivery) or 96-hours (for cesarean section delivery). State laws like Act 81 support the federal mandate, require carrier compliance, extend the number of covered days without actual enrollment on the policy, recognize both parents as potential subscribers for available coverage, etc. § 54.9811-1 Standards relating to benefits for mothers and newborns Title 26, Chapter 1, Subchapter D, Part 54, Section 54.9811-1) and Pennsylvania Code, § 89.201, Subchapter F, Coverage for Newborn Children (PA Act 81)	

SUMMARY OF EFFECTIVE PRACTICE: The premise that there should be a uniform approach as it relates to newborns and maximizing available primary coverage; i.e. if there were to be some model DRA language that states could adopt within their own state "DRA" language. It was indicated in our vendor's opinion; PA has proper language (PA Act 81) as it relates to the project being introduced to the carrier community. Essentially, the project was a result of learning more about the PA Act 81 language through the Pennsylvania Department of Public Welfare (DPW) inquiry to our vendor, which led to a national project approach on behalf of all vendor clients. A process was developed to identify newborns with available primary coverage through a parent subscriber policy. Once billing of claims to carriers began, leverage from both Act 81 and the Federal mandates lead to a carrier education campaign covering this "Newborn" population across the country and within the timely filing limits of the state's DRA language. The DPW provides eligibility and paid claims files to the vendor. The process begins with the vendor identifying date of service equals date of birth, a claim has been paid by the Medicaid program, identifying other primary coverage that is available using data matching algorithms in conjunction with the National Eligibility Database. Added quality checks to confirm parent/dependent relationship are used. Once primary coverage is confirmed for one of the parents associated with the newborn, paid claims are billed to the primary carrier for reimbursement back to the Medicaid agency. The DPW collects payments and has generated more than $1.2 million in recoveries for PA DPW to date. There is still additional follow up and education to be performed with the carrier community. As this continued claims identification, coverage confirmation, claims billings and carrier education occur, our vendor anticipates ongoing recoveries from the $9 million+ in PA newborn claims that have been billed to date, as well as continued recovery opportunity, as newborns with available primary coverage are identified. This project can also lead to potential HIPP referrals for those cost-effective scenarios, since the ultimate goal should be to enroll the newborn in available commercial coverage to ensure that the Medicaid program remains the payer of last resort and cost-avoided savings are maximized.
SPECIAL FACTORS THAT SUPPORT THE EFFECTIVE PRACTICE: (Ex: State Law, Case Law, Data Exchange Agreements, Data Systems, Contractor Use, etc.) Pennsylvania has a contractor perform data exchange and recovery services. § 54.9811-1 Standards relating to benefits for mothers and newborns Title 26, Chapter 1, Subchapter D, Part 54, Section 54.9811-1) and Pennsylvania Code,

§ 89.201, Subchapter F, Coverage for Newborn Children (PA Act 81)
FOR MORE INFORMATION, CONTACT: Carole Procope | TPL Director (Name and Title, Phone Number, Email Address) Department of Public Welfare | Bureau of Program Integrity 116 East Azalea Drive | Harrisburg, PA 17110-3594 Phone: 717.705.8234 | Fax: 717.772.6553 www.dpw.state.pa.us

TEXAS

ISSUE: Denials from third parties for procedural reasons	
IN THE RESPONDING STATE, THIS ISSUE: ____CURRENTLY OCCURS OR HAS OCCURRED: ____VERY FREQUENTLY __X__OFTEN ENOUGH TO REQUIRE CORRECTION ____ INFREQUENTLY ____ DOESN'T OCCUR OR HASN'T OCCURRED	***EFFECT OF THE PRACTICE:*** ____RESOLVED THE ISSUE FULLY ____RESOLVED THE ISSUE PARTIALLY (*Indicate what was resolved and what remains in the Summary below.*) __X__RESOLVED TEMPORARILY WITH A WORKAROUND PROCESS
WHY DOES THIS ISSUE OCCUR? Texas found that payers are denying our Medicaid reclamation claims for procedural reasons. To mitigate the loss of recovery dollars, we directed our vendor to create a Denials Team to manually review these third party claim denials and determine if they could be rebilled for payment.	
SUMMARY OF EFFECTIVE PRACTICE: Our vendor established the Denials Team in 2009 which is responsible for researching the Explanation of Benefits (EOBs) in order to identify claims denied inappropriately. Claims found to have been denied inappropriately are appealed to the carrier. Not only has this process resulted in increased recoveries from the insurance carriers it has also lead to provider recoupments in situations where we discovered that the providers received payment from Medicaid and from the insurance carrier as well.	
SPECIAL FACTORS THAT SUPPORT THE EFFECTIVE PRACTICE:	

(Ex: State Law, Case Law, Data Exchange Agreements, Data Systems, Contractor Use, etc.) Since the creation of the Denials team in May 2009 they have recovered $39,612,696.25 in this one category alone. See the breakout below for all denial recoveries and recoupments by State Fiscal Year (SFY) from 2009 - present. SFY 2009 $458,746.00 (5 of 12 months) SFY 2010 $ 1,632,707.00 SFY 2011 $ 8,977,959.00 SFY 2012 $13,051.780.00 SFY 2013 $13,032,474.66 SFYTD 2014 $ 2,459,029.59
FOR MORE INFORMATION, CONTACT: (Name and Title, Phone Number, Email Address) Diane Broadhurst, TPL Manager, 512-491-5638, diane.broadhurst@hhsc.state.tx.us

TEXAS

ISSUE: Cooperation from pharmacy benefit managersand other entities	
IN THE RESPONDING STATE, THIS ISSUE: __X__CURRENTLY OCCURS OR HAS OCCURRED: ____ VERY FREQUENTLY __X__OFTEN ENOUGH TO REQUIRE CORRECTION ____ INFREQUENTLY ____ DOESN'T OCCUR OR HASN'T OCCURRED	*EFFECT OF THE PRACTICE:* __X__RESOLVED THE ISSUE FULLY ____RESOLVED THE ISSUE PARTIALLY (*Indicate what was resolved and what remains in the Summary below.*) ____RESOLVED TEMPORARILY WITH A WORKAROUND PROCESS
WHY DOES THIS ISSUE OCCUR? Some insurance carriers/pharmacy benefit managers/third party administrators operating in the State of Texas did not want to perform data matches with the State Medicaid Agency in a timely fashion.	
SUMMARY OF EFFECTIVE PRACTICE: Texas statute in place prior to 2007 only required these entities to perform data	

matches once every six (6) months. However, in 2007, a new statute was implemented that required entities doing business in the State of Texas to enter into an agreement with the Health and Human Services Commission (HHSC). This agreement and the associated processes are known as the Billing Coordination System (BCS). One of the provisions within the BCS statute requires that any entity that holds a permit, license, or certificate of authority issued by a regulatory agency of the state must allow HHSC access to databases to allow for the identification of other payers. If the other entity does not allow access, then the entity is subject to an administrative penalty or other sanction as provided by the law applicable to the permit, license, or certificate of authority for a violation by the entity of a rule adopted under this section. The initial BCS legislation was only applicable to Fee for Service (FFS) and Primary Care Case Management (PCCM) services. In the following two legislative sessions (2009 & 2011), additional provisions were added to the BCS statute and the requirement has been expanded to include all Medicaid and non-Medicaid programs overseen by HHSC. Texas is currently working on revising the carrier agreements to include not only medical insurance carriers, but pharmacy benefit managers (PBMs), long term care (LTC) carriers, and third party administrators (TPAs). The BCS Carrier Agreements have resulted in HHSC's ability to match more frequently (biweekly/monthly/quarterly) with carriers which allows for more timely TPL identification for purposes of cost avoidance and cost recovery. In addition, with the expansion of managed care in Texas, these agreements will allow HHSC the ability to take on sole responsibility for TPL identification and share it with both our FFS Fiscal Agent and with the MCO's allowing us the ability to set performance standards and service level agreements for those vendors in order for HHSC to ensure that Texas is in compliance with federal and state TPL requirements.
SPECIAL FACTORS THAT SUPPORT THE EFFECTIVE PRACTICE: (Ex: State Law, Case Law, Data Exchange Agreements, Data Systems, Contractor Use, etc.) Texas Government Code Chapter 531- Health and Human Services Commission, Section 531.02413-Billing Coordination System
FOR MORE INFORMATION, CONTACT: (Name and Title, Phone Number, Email Address) Diane Broadhurst, TPL Manager, 512-491-5638, diane.broadhurst@hhsc.state.tx.us

WASHINGTON

<table>
<tr><td colspan="2">ISSUE:Dept. of Transportation data match</td></tr>
<tr><td>IN THE RESPONDING STATE, THIS ISSUE:

____CURRENTLY OCCURS OR HAS OCCURRED:
___X_VERY FREQUENTLY
____OFTEN ENOUGH TO REQUIRE CORRECTION
____INFREQUENTLY
____DOESN'T OCCUR OR HASN'T OCCURRED</td><td>EFFECT OF THE PRACTICE:

____RESOLVED THE ISSUE FULLY
__X__RESOLVED THE ISSUE PARTIALLY (Indicate what was resolved and what remains in the Summary below.)
____RESOLVED TEMPORARILY WITH A WORKAROUND PROCESS</td></tr>
<tr><td colspan="2">WHY DOES THIS ISSUE OCCUR? n/a</td></tr>
<tr><td colspan="2">SUMMARY OF EFFECTIVE PRACTICE:

A data match between Washington State's Department of Social and Health Services (DSHS), Coordination of Benefits Section's, Casualty Unit and Department of Transportation was established in 2006. The purpose of the match is to compare names and dates of birth of Medicaid clients with the Washington State Patrol motor vehicle accident records. A report is produced and staff validate whetherthird party liability is available. Prior to this exchange we relied primarily on attorney contacts, paid claims, and diagnosis based Treatment Questionnaires as resources for case managers.

Information on all traffic accidents in the State of Washington is uploaded to our system and matched against Medicaid clients on a weekly basis. Staff members examine claims data to determine if there is potential recovery. The purpose is to catch the Motor Vehicle Accidents (MVAs) early, before the insurance companies have a chance to settle. MVAs comprise 75% of our Casualty Unit's caseload.

One drawback has been that in some cases we are too early...the claims have not been submitted yet. Providers have 365 days to submit a claim and we are looking for claims data prior to then. Our Information Technology resources are limited, however, we'd like to develop an automated recheck process...60/90/120 days sometime in the future to alleviate this problem.</td></tr>
</table>

DATE SPREAD	TOTALS	Purge Hits	WSP SEARCHS	PENDINGCREATED
2/1/13-3/8/13	320	21	19	12
2/1/13-3/15/13	481	21	20	9
2/1/13-3/22/13	324	14	10	8
3/1/13-3/29/13	327	20	14	7
3/1/13-4/5/13	302	19	15	8
3/1/13-4/12/13	285	8	8	5
3/1/13-4/19/13	358	11	8	4
4/1/13-4/26/13	383	13	10	7
4/1/13-5/3/13	512	12	11	8
4/1/13-5/10/13	524	16	13	9
4/1/13-5/17/13	427	18	13	10
5/1/13-5/24/13	507	16	14	9
5/1/13-5/31/13	381	14	12	7
5/1/13-6/7/13	701	28	23	18
5/1/13-6/14/13	1053	17	15	7
6/1/13-6/21/13	2196	36	27	13
6/1/13-6/28/13	1027	17	12	10
6/1/13-7/5/13	122	0	0	0
6/1/13-7/12/13	1056	10	9	4

KEY:
Date Spread: Transaction Dates that collision reports are filed into the DMV system
Purge Hits: Medicaid claims occurring close to the date of the auto accident WSP Searches:
The Washington State Patrol Collision record searches
Pending Created: Identification of previously unknown cases

SPECIAL FACTORS THAT SUPPORT THE EFFECTIVE PRACTICE:

(Ex: State Law, Case Law, Data Exchange Agreements, Data Systems, Contractor Use, etc.)
Originally, an interagency agreement was established between the Department of Transportation and (now) Washington State Health Care Authority's Coordination of Benefits Section to enable the transfer of a monthly disk. This process evolved into a web-based application which narrows the search to just those accidents involving Medicaid clients. This process is a requirement in our State Plan.

FOR MORE INFORMATION, CONTACT:

(Name and Title, Phone Number, Email Address)

Andy Renggli, Coordination of Benefits Section Manager andy.renggli@hca.wa.gov (360) 725-1207

WASHINGTON

ISSUE: Payer Initiated Eligibility/Benefit (PIE) Transaction	
IN THE RESPONDING STATE, THIS ISSUE: ____CURRENTLY OCCURS OR HAS OCCURRED: ____VERY FREQUENTLY ____OFTEN ENOUGH TO REQUIRE CORRECTION ____INFREQUENTLY ____DOESN'T OCCUR OR HASN'T OCCURRED	*EFFECT OF THE PRACTICE:* ____RESOLVED THE ISSUE FULLY ____RESOLVED THE ISSUE PARTIALLY (Indicate what was resolved and what remains in the Summary below.) ____RESOLVED TEMPORARILY WITH A WORKAROUND PROCESS
WHY DOES THIS ISSUE OCCUR? Efficient methods for exchanging clients' eligibility for health coverage and their associated benefits are a continuous, on-going need in Coordination of Benefits.	
SUMMARY OF EFFECTIVE PRACTICE: WA State Medicaid has recently published the Payer Initiated Eligibility (PIE) transaction guide at http://www.hca.wa.gov/medicaid/hipaa/Documents/wammis cg pie 271-501007052013version1.pdf.	
The purpose of this transaction guide is to assist payers information to State Medicaid programs. The Centers Payer Initiated Eligibility/Benefit (PIE) Transaction which The Guide focuses on the exchange of data from payers geographic areas to be covered by the transaction and delivery will be addressed in the trading partner agreement. The Washington State Medicaid Management Information ready to accept the PIE transaction. in providing health plan eligibility and coverage for Medicare & Medicaid Services developed the can be used to meet the DRA requirements. to Medicaid agencies. Agreement regarding the schedule and frequency of transaction System (MMIS) named ProviderOne is now	
SPECIAL FACTORS THAT SUPPORT THE EFFECTIVE PRACTICE: (Ex: State Law, Case Law, Data Exchange Agreements, Data Systems, Contractor Use, etc.) The PIE transaction was developed to comply with both the federal Deficit	

Reduction Act of 2005 and Washington State Substitute House Bill 1826 (http://www.leg.wa.gov/pub/billinfo/2007-08/pdf/bills/house%20passed%20legislature/ 1826-s.pl.pdf
Federal law requires States to identify and obtain payment from third party entities that are legally responsible to pay claims primary to Medicaid. To enhance States' abilities to identify legally liable third parties, the Deficit Reduction Act of 2005 (DRA) required States to pass laws imposing requirements on health plans, as a condition of doing business in the State, to provide plan eligibility information to the State. The Payer Initiated Eligibility/Benefit (PIE) Transaction will be used to provide Washington State Medicaid with a listing that identifies plan members' eligibility for health coverage and their associated benefits. Of course the same transaction format can be used by all states and all carriers. The PIE Transaction was developed to deliver membership and benefit information in one single, unsolicited transaction. The PIE Transaction uses the same identifiers as the ASC X12 271 response transaction and therefore mirrors the format of the 271 transaction. The purpose of the transaction guide is to provide a standardized format for the PIE Transaction information. The information supplied on the PIE Transaction is to be as comprehensive as possible, with beginning and end dates and including other coverage, if available. The provided information will be used to match to the Washington State's Provider One database. For this purpose, a required key data element is the Social Security Number. If the Social Security Number is not available, other key identifiers may be used.
FOR MORE INFORMATION, CONTACT: (Name and Title, Phone Number, Email Address) Andy Renggli, Coordination of Benefits Section Manager andy.renggli@hca.wa.gov (360) 725-1207

INDEX

P

Q

R

S

T

U

V

W

Y